Standards and Ethics for Counselling in Action

SAGE Counselling in Action

is a bestselling series of short, practical introductions designed for students and trainees. Covering theory and practice, the books are core texts for many courses, both in counselling and other professions such as nursing, social work and teaching.

Books in the series include:

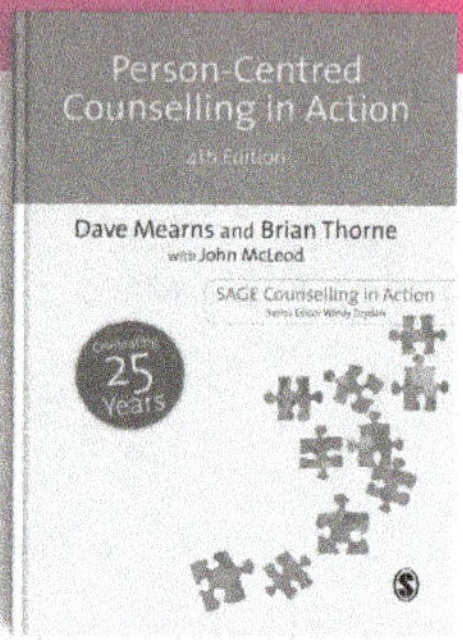

978-1-4462-5253-6

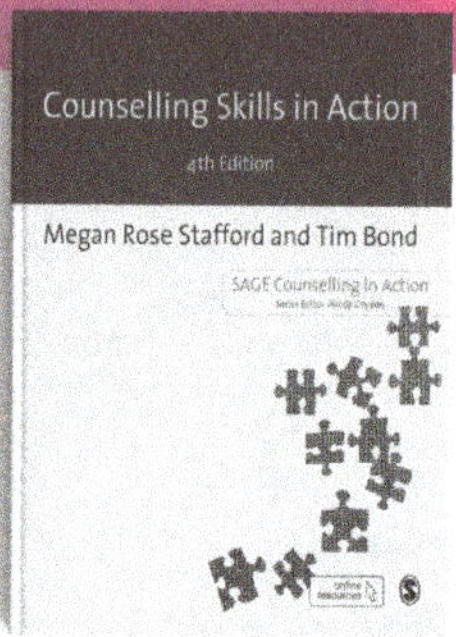

978-1-4739-9818-6

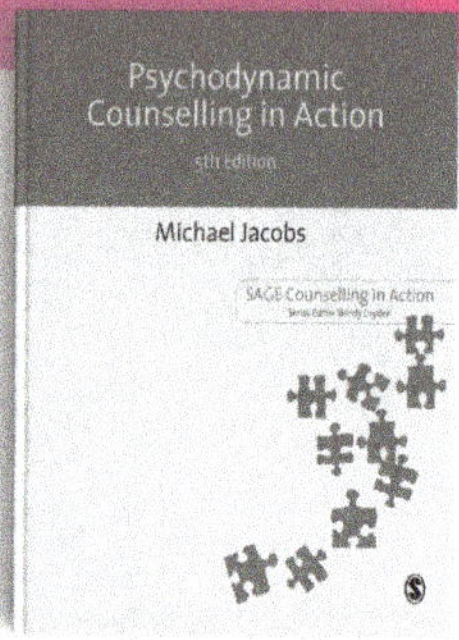

978-1-4739-9816-2

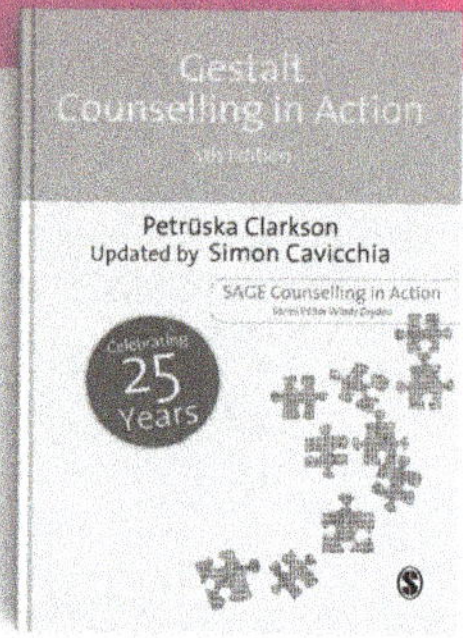

978-1-4462-1128-1

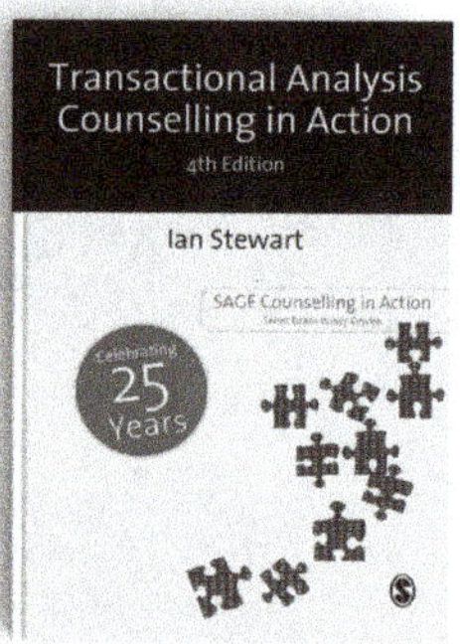

978-1-4462-5328-1

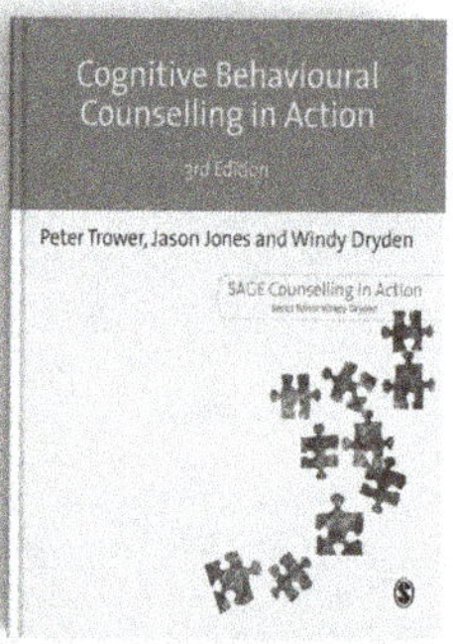

978-1-4739-1369-1

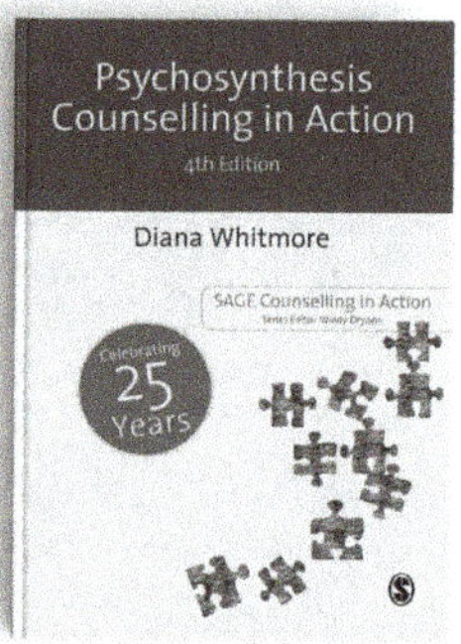

978-1-4462-5293-2

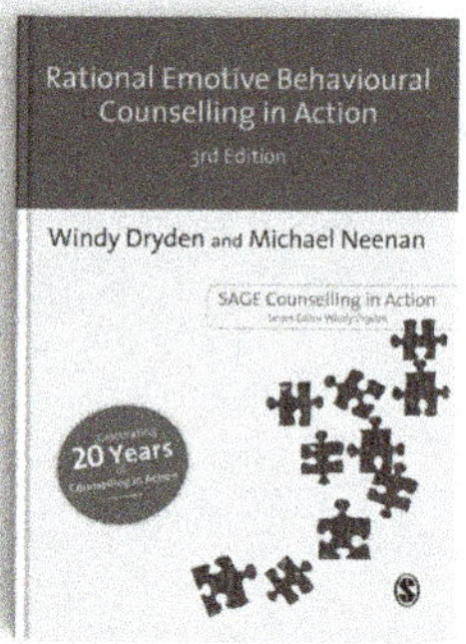

978-1-4129-0213-7

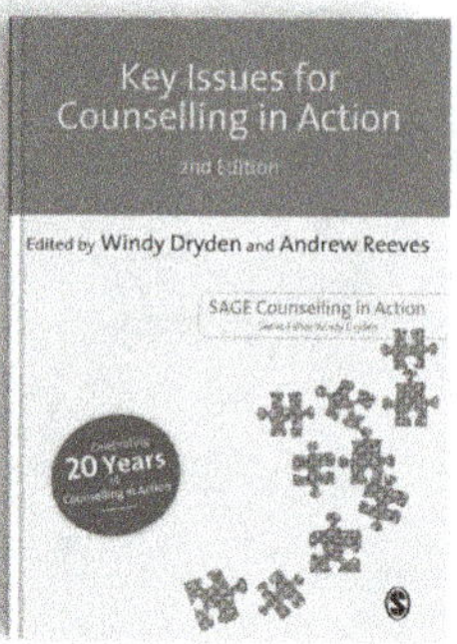

978-1-4129-4699-5

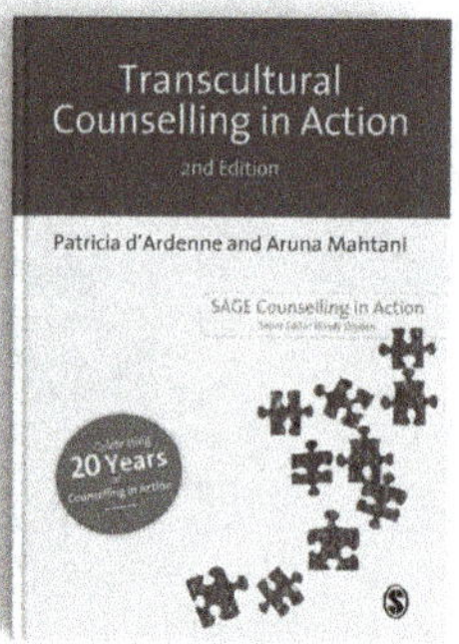

978-0-7619-6315-8

Standards and Ethics for Counselling in Action

5th Edition

Andrew Reeves & Tim Bond

SAGE Counselling in Action
Series Editor Windy Dryden

SAGE

Los Angeles | London | New Delhi
Singapore | Washington DC | Melbourne

SAGE

Los Angeles | London | New Delhi
Singapore | Washington DC | Melbourne

SAGE Publications Ltd
1 Oliver's Yard
55 City Road
London EC1Y 1SP

SAGE Publications Inc.
2455 Teller Road
Thousand Oaks, California 91320

SAGE Publications India Pvt Ltd
B 1/I 1 Mohan Cooperative Industrial Area
Mathura Road
New Delhi 110 044

SAGE Publications Asia-Pacific Pte Ltd
3 Church Street
#10-04 Samsung Hub
Singapore 049483

Editor: Susannah Trefgarne
Assistant editor: Ruth Lilly
Assistant editor, digital: Sunita Patel
Production editor: Rachel Burrows
Marketing manager: Dilhara Attygalle
Cover design: Naomi Robinson
Typeset by: C&M Digitals (P) Ltd, Chennai, India

Library of Congress Control Number: 2020947335

British Library Cataloguing in Publication data

A catalogue record for this book is available from the British Library

ISBN 978-1-5264-5886-5
ISBN 978-1-5264-5887-2 (pbk)

Contents

About the Authors

Andrew Reeves is an Associate Professor in the Counselling Professions and Mental Health, a Senior BACP Accredited Counsellor/Psychotherapist and a Registered Social Worker. He is a past Chair of the British Association for Counselling and Psychotherapy, a Fellow of BACP and a Senior Fellow of Advance HE. He has published extensively on working in counselling and psychotherapy, and particularly in working with risk in a range of organizational settings. He is past Editor-in-Chief of the journal *Counselling and Psychotherapy Research* and has a long-standing commitment to ethics in the counselling professions, including in writing and research.

Tim Bond is an Emeritus Professor of the University of Bristol and Visiting Professor to the University of Malta. He has a long-standing commitment to researching and writing about professional ethics for the talking therapies and promoting mental wellbeing. He has been a consultant to the British Association for Counselling and Psychotherapy on professional ethics and standards, a member of the Ethics Committee for the British Psychological Society and the Executive Council of the International Association for Counselling. He is a registered member of BACP and provides counselling supervision and training workshops.

Acknowledgements

This is the first edition of this text to be jointly authored and we are delighted to have had the opportunity to work with each other in its production. As such, it with enormous thanks to each other for mutual guidance, support, encouragement and the opportunity itself.

Once again, we have both greatly enjoyed working with a team from SAGE, particularly Susannah Trefgarne, Ruth Lilly and Rachel Burrows.

We are indebted to the legal and ethical expertise of Ba Mitchels with whom Tim has co-authored many books and valued many discussions about ethical and legal issues.

We are particularly grateful to the counsellors and therapist who generously agreed to take on roles in the video clips that accompany this book. They are Leanne Hoffman, Emily Holt, Anne Stokes and Sarah Williams. They brought what is exemplary in the videos from their own expertise and experience. Whatever is questionable is the result of instructions given to them by Tim to encourage viewers to reflect on ethics and standards. Further to acknowledge the actors Tor Clark and James Messer, Phil Desmeules as Actor Liaison, Emily Smail Runner, Nic Giammetta Sound, David Smail Camera and Jo Sutton Director.

Families, friends and good colleagues are always critical in the development of books such as this. It is they who have accompanied us on our respective journeys that have been so critical in developing our world views and the sense we have made of the ethical opportunities and challenges that have come our way; they have, without doubt, been figural in shaping the position we have taken in our writing here. For Andrew, huge thanks go to Diane, Adam, Katie and Emily for – once again – not rolling their eyes but rather smiling encouragingly when I mention I have another writing project on the go. To Hadyn Williams, for suggesting to Tim that I might be a worthy co-author on this book that has meant so much to me over the years in my own practice and, of course, to Tim – for agreeing to Hadyn's suggestion. Tim does not recall the detail of examining my doctoral thesis many years before this point (but I do), but now to have an opportunity to work alongside him has been an honour and pleasure in equal measure.

In each previous edition I, Tim, have sought to acknowledge the impact of writing these books on my family. There is always a tension because writing is largely solitary and sometimes leaves me absent-minded, even when I am trying to be sociable and enjoy the people around me. Jan, as always, has offered words of wisdom and encouragement as we navigate busy professional lives with the joys and demands of family life. We are conscious of how each edition has marked a different stage in the lives of our children. At the time of the first edition Sam was a 'bump' eagerly awaited by his toddler sister Zoe. Now both are young adults building their own trajectories through life – except when interrupted by me for technical advice on computing and new technology! However, some habits have passed through the generations. They are both interested in ethics and quick to spot any of my ethical failings in our lives together – often accompanied by lively discussions and laughter. Their questions and challenges are a constant reminder to me that ethics are about how we live together as people and face the challenges of life.

We are writing this latest edition in the midst of a COVID-19 viral pandemic. One of the consequences of the challenges posed by this particular coronavirus is that everyone is faced with ethical choices that involve balancing what is good for us as individuals and what is good for the community. Ethics are no longer just the reference points for resolving moral choices within professions but have become more consciously part of everyday life. The ethics in this book provide us with a language and ideas about how to help everyone make the best ethical choices for their circumstances.

Online Resources

This Fifth Edition of *Standards and Ethics for Counselling in Action* is supported by online resources to aid study and assist in teaching, which are available at https://study.sagepub.com/reevesandbond

Videos: Watch more than 40 videos, including videos of counselling scenarios illustrating ethical issues in practice and videos of the authors discussing key ethical topics and dilemmas. Each video comes with questions that help you to extend your knowledge of a topic. To access the exclusive SAGE Videos, please see the code on the inside front cover of your textbook. If you have purchased the eBook from Amazon or another online retailer, please email DigitalContent@sagepub.co.uk with the subject line 'Access Code Required' and we will assist further.

Further reading: Access a wealth of free online journal articles on the website. Use these readings to help deepen your knowledge and reinforce your learning of key topics.

List of Videos

Part I

The Background

1

Introduction

Chapter Overview

Good practice that benefits clients requires an understanding of **standards** and **ethics** as the basis for earning a client's **trust**. Key terms are defined with examples of common sources of misunderstanding. This chapter considers positive **ethical standards** and examples of the poor practice these are designed to counteract. It concludes with the basic question 'Why be ethical?'

Key words

standards, ethics, **morals**, ethical standards, trust

Counselling ethics do not stand still. New **issues** emerge. New practices develop. Our clients' expectations change. The regulatory and legal context of our work evolves. In this fifth edition we have updated the information in the light of this changing world, recognizing the impact of social changes in which counselling is contextualized, such as the #BlackLivesMatter and #MeToo movements, as well as the changes forced upon the nature and delivery of counselling during the

COVID-19 pandemic. Ethics continue to provide an imperative for the delivery of high standards of practice in the counselling professions and the need to evolve in the light of those changes too. These will be further explored with additional features: *Pause for Reflection* and *Social Justice in Context*. This new edition works to consider those standards and ethics in action.

How to Use This Book

This book is intended to be practical, and the hope is that many people will want to read it from cover to cover. Contents have been organized so that the logical structure of counselling ethics and **standards** of practice becomes apparent progressively throughout the book. However, when working with clients there is not always the time for extensive reading when information or inspiration is needed; we tend to dip into books looking for specific topics. In keeping this in mind, related issues have been grouped together into chapters. The Index at the end of the book is designed to help you locate passages on specific topics.

We begin by explaining why standards and ethics are important and describe the contribution and role of the British Association for Counselling and Psychotherapy (BACP) and other national organizations in developing standards and ethics for counsellors. The second chapter considers the fundamental question 'What is counselling?' because the answer is so important if we are to decide which matters fall within the scope of counselling and which more properly belong to other roles and are therefore covered by different systems of ethics and practice. The third chapter provides a review of the main sources of material for the production of standards and ethics. An ethical framework for the application of these sources to counselling is proposed in Chapter 4. All the following chapters take a theme or closely related set of issues and explore it in more detail in ways which we hope will be useful to practitioners. It is part of the nature of this subject that, in the last resort, every practitioner has to assess each situation for themselves and reach a personal decision, so the last chapter proposes a procedure for assessing and resolving **dilemmas** about standards and ethics.

Concerns about Standards and Ethics

In preparing this new edition, we have drawn on many years' experience as members of various ethics and professional conduct committees, and both as former Chairs of

BACP. Some of the issues that cause counsellors most concern are misunderstandings about the following.

What counselling is, or is not, and the results of this

- *Inappropriate referrals*: 'I want you to counsel Brian off this course', 'Would you see Beryl and counsel her to take early retirement because we need to reorganize the distribution of work in her office?'.
- *Inappropriate expectations of the counsellor in relation to* ***confidentiality***: 'I wouldn't have asked John to see you if I had realized you wouldn't tell me what he said to you.'
- *Confusion among counsellors about the* ***limitations*** *of confidentiality*: 'Am I obliged to report all instances of suspected child abuse?'
- *Questioning the opportunities and limitations of counselling*: 'Wouldn't it be better to intervene to stop people being emotionally traumatized by the bully rather than continuing to patch up the casualties?'
- *Adapting ethics to different cultural contexts*: 'How far should I adapt my counselling ethics to meet the needs of clients from different cultures and social contexts?'
- *Adapting ethics to new methods of delivering counselling*: 'How should I adapt to providing counselling using electronic technologies like webcam, email and texting?'

Counselling supervision

- *Confusion between counselling* ***supervision*** *and* ***accountability*** *to line management*: 'As your line manager I am accountable for your work. I don't want someone else confusing matters', or 'No other staff get independent supervision and support so I find it difficult to see why counsellors should be any different.'
- *The need for ongoing long-term supervision*: 'Surely you must be out of your probationary period by now. I can't see why you still need supervision.'

The need for training

- *Confusion over levels of* ***competence*** *requiring corresponding levels of training*: 'We all counsel, don't we? Surely three days' training is more than enough.'
- *The possibility of creating instant experts in counselling*: 'Here are two books on counselling. I want you to read them this weekend and become the counsellor on Monday.'

Comments such as these are often heard from counsellors in schools, colleges, hospitals, social services, employee assistance programmes, pastoral care, **voluntary** organizations and private practice.

These and many other issues are the subject matter of this book.

The importance of standards and ethics

Counselling depends on clients being able to **trust** their counsellors. They trust their feelings of vulnerability to someone who is committed to using their knowledge and skills to act in the best interests of their clients. Professions honour and protect this trust by setting standards for their practitioners and expecting them to act ethically. Good standards and ethical practice provide the best possible conditions for clients to discuss freely whatever is causing them concern and for the counsellor to work therapeutically.

Standards define the essential safeguards and required level of expertise to provide a safe and effective service to clients. Standards typically define the level of training, continuing professional development, supervision, **insurance** and service delivery in terms of competence and good conduct. Failing to meet minimum or fundamental standards is a serious matter. It may result in disciplinary or fitness to practise hearings against individual counsellors held by employers or by professional bodies. Where whole services fail to meet the minimum or fundamental standard, their continued existence is called into question. Following a major lapse in standards in healthcare resulting in additional suffering and the premature deaths of vulnerable elderly patients, the Francis Report (2013) distinguished three levels of standards:

- *Fundamental standards of* ***safety*** *and quality*: the level below which a service ought not to be offered because it exposes patients or clients to avoidable harm.
- *Enhanced quality standards*: the level that the funding will support above fundamental standards and can be achieved by improvements in professionalism or management.
- *Developmental standards*: the level to which a service might aspire in the longer term out of a commitment to progress and excellence.

From a client's point of view, standards imply a system of quality control and assurance that extends beyond their individual counsellor and that this counsellor is both supported by and accountable to others for the work undertaken. Clients often see standards as a source of reassurance. Standards exist in the general awareness of many clients as something they expect of a professional service. Even when these are not fully understood by clients, their existence provides some reassurance as they build a relationship with a counsellor who will often be a stranger to them. Standards may also be seen as a point of reference to assess or resolve any difficulties that may arise. When something is claimed to be a 'standard', this implies that the standard has been set on the basis of evidence about its beneficial effects, that it is supported by a professional knowledge, that it is measureable or observable so that whether it is being achieved can be evaluated, and that there is a body responsible for overseeing that the standard is being satisfied. The body for overseeing standards in the first instance might be the agency delivering the service, a professional organization, and ultimately the registration or regulatory body for the profession. The person in the front line of clients' awareness of standards will be their counsellor and many clients will look no further when all is going well.

Ethics provide ideas and terminology for considering what is morally good or bad and how to distinguish good from bad. Ethics and **morals** are often regarded as meaning the same things in everyday speech. Frequently this use of both terms interchangeably does not matter because the focus is not on the precise meaning but on distinguishing good from bad. However, there is a distinction that may be useful in professional ethics. Morals are the norms we acquire from our **culture** and social background. They inform how people coexist. Morals may be treated as unquestioned assumptions or subject to careful consideration, particularly during periods of social change. The **law** is a form of enforceable morals that have the weight of the national system of government behind them. 'Morals' and 'morality' are therefore all-encompassing terms that include any claims to what is good or bad. This all-encompassing use of morals can be distinguished from ethics which are the result of a careful and conscious consideration of what is good or bad and the distinction between good and bad can be explained.

Professional ethics are an applied form of ethics that are specific to particular roles and contexts. This distinction is useful to draw attention to why some issues may be approached differently in everyday life in comparison to the applicable professional ethics. For example, it is morally desirable for friends to offer help to each other spontaneously and in an open-ended way, but counsellors are expected to offer help on the basis of agreed terms and conditions, typically presented in the form of a **contract**. Strong emotional and sexual relationships are generally considered a moral good between unattached adults, whereas sexual relationships between counsellors and clients are considered ethically bad and forbidden. Good-natured gossip in everyday life is arguably morally and socially beneficial in that it strengthens the bonds between people, may provide useful learning opportunities about social living, and enlivens lives. In contrast, **respect** for the **privacy** of clients and protecting their confidentiality is a major ethical concern in counselling and arguably one of its distinctive ethical preoccupations.

Establishing a distinction between morals and ethics is also helpful in responding to social diversity. For example, there are many instances of deeply held ethnic practices or religious beliefs that may impose strict limitations on contacts between genders, sexual behaviours in opposite or same-sex relationships, relationships outside a faith or ethnic group, and social or dietary requirements. The moral expectations within the applicable community are clear, but should counselling be restricted to people who conform to these expectations? Ought counselling to be offered more widely to people who struggle to meet these expectations or disagree with them? This is a question of how professional ethics ought to relate to a prevailing morality or respond to the sometimes conflicted relationships between different moral communities. Sometimes it is helpful to re-examine whether prevailing moral assumptions have been incorporated in professional ethics which, on closer examination, restrict the usefulness of counselling for people from different moral communities. Counselling has largely developed in cultures with a strong sense of individualism, but how should counsellors work respectfully with people who have a strong sense of collective **identity** around an extended family or network of extended families with a tribe or clan? The ethics of responding to social diversity are considered in more depth in Chapter 12. Making a distinction between morality and ethics makes it easier to identify potential points of difference and difficulty and recognizes that public morals and professional ethics are established in different ways and serve different purposes.

There are certain types of difficulties that have been reported by clients with sufficient frequency over the fifty or more years of counselling that their remedy is to identify a positive ethical standard that would redress the concern and support good practice. The following list presents a positive ethical example followed by the sorts of issues that have breached that standard. These examples of bad or poor practice could have been prevented if the counsellor had observed the ethical standard:

- *Being **trustworthy***: counsellors who have broken promises in what they offered or in the management of client confidences, leaving clients feeling betrayed.
- *A counsellor setting aside personal interests and putting the client's interests first*: information provided in counselling used to benefit the counsellor financially or emotionally by having early knowledge of property coming onto the market or forming a relationship with the client's recently estranged partner; conflicts of interest concealed or not declared.

- *A clear understanding of what to expect*: muddled beginnings where the client is unclear about what they are committing to, any liabilities for payments, or how confidentiality will be managed and protected.
- *The client respected as a person*: the counsellor prejudiced against the client either as person or as representative of a social group or way of living of which the counsellor disapproves, or the counsellor pursuing a personal religious- or value-based agenda regardless of a client's deeply held **values**.
- *Maintaining* ***boundaries*** *in relationships that support the counselling*: counsellors forming relationships with clients or their circles of friends to resolve their own loneliness or meet sexual desires; failing to consider how boundaries will be managed if the client and counsellor meet outside counselling sessions in other roles or settings, whether planned or accidentally.
- *Being competent*: the counsellor offering services for which they lack adequate knowledge, skills or organizational ability, working without appropriate supervision or adequate continuing professional development.
- *Working with* ***integrity***: the counsellor is dishonest about their qualifications or experience or other matters important to the client or the profession.
- *Being accountable to the client*: confused or inconsistent communications about how the counselling has been delivered and why; poor record keeping when **records** were expected as good practice or promised; concealing a mistake from a client rather than alerting them, attempting to minimize any harm, and apologizing.
- *Well-managed endings*: the client is unprepared for the ending and left feeling abandoned and unsupported to meet the counsellor's convenience or needs.
- *Protecting the reputation of counselling*: behaving so badly in or outside the counselling relationship that the reputation of counselling has been undermined in the eyes of the public.

Sadly this list is not fully comprehensive of all the examples of poor or bad practice that we have been aware of involving a variety of professional bodies, and some of the most serious have often appeared to involve counsellors working without any professional membership or organization to call them to account. The list includes some examples where clients have been seriously hurt or damaged psychologically or they consider that their reputation has been damaged in the eyes of others. As professional conduct hearings are increasingly open and report findings against counsellors, it is informative to periodically review the background and outcomes of cases reported by professional bodies like the British Association for Counselling and Psychotherapy (BACP), fitness-to-practise hearings against counselling psychologists by the Health and Care Professions Council (HCPC), or similar proceedings in other organizations or countries. There is interesting **research** into what makes talking therapy safe from the clients' point of view, resulting in some positive recommendations.

Whilst not understating the seriousness of some these examples for the clients affected, it is important to emphasize the importance of a positive ethical commitment. For every example of poor practice, there are many more counsellors who have been deeply committed to being ethical. There is a strong culture of altruism and compassion that motivates most counsellors. Nonetheless, good intent is necessary but not sufficient to do good. We all benefit from reminding ourselves about how things can go wrong and why it matters that we are committed to being ethical.

Why Be Ethical?

Unless counselling is provided on an ethical basis, it ceases to serve any useful purpose. Clients will usually seek counselling because they are troubled or vulnerable; they wish to be sure that the primary concern of the counselling is to help them to achieve a greater sense of control and wellbeing in their lives and that counselling is not being used in order to serve some other purpose. This means that counselling, by its very nature, needs to be an ethical relationship.

However, clients are not usually well informed about the **ethical standards** of counselling, so they are more likely to judge the ethical basis of their counselling by assessing the personal integrity of the counsellor. This is much more familiar ground. Every day, all of us are engaged in assessing the trustworthiness of the people we meet. One of the first concerns of a client at the start of counselling is 'How far can I trust this person to be my counsellor?' Typically, it is assumed that if the counsellor appears to have personal integrity, then the ethical standards that they apply to their counselling will be of a similar level. By definition, trust always involves a leap of faith, which overrides a lack of information and ignorance in order to place confidence in a person or system. This is a major step for many clients. Some will manage the risk by testing out the counsellor on less serious issues before disclosing the real concern. Others will be so driven by the urgency of the situation or their distress that the problem will come tumbling out before they have sat down. In either situation, this act of trust comes at a time of considerable vulnerability for the client and gives the counsellor considerable power over them for good or harm. This is why the counsellor's personal commitment to being ethical is so vital. One person's vulnerability creates a corresponding obligation for the other in their exercise of power and professional expertise.

Without the act of trust, counselling is impossible. Sufficient trust needs to be present to enable clients to participate with appropriate frankness and active commitment. Counselling is not like a medical procedure that can take place on a passive or anaesthetized patient. It requires the active participation and engagement of clients made possible by a relationship of trust. Establishing a high level of trust in the counselling is considered to be so fundamental that it is the primary principle in some constructions of counselling ethics (Bond, 2006, 2007). It is also the basis of the legal protection of confidences imparted in counselling in many jurisdictions, including English law. Even when trust is not regarded as the primary ethical requirement for counselling, it is always high on the list of ethical priorities. Different approaches to the construction of counselling ethics are considered in Chapters 3 and 4. The one thing that unites the people who developed these approaches is the conviction that a commitment to being ethical is the best way of protecting the interests of the client and enhancing the reputation of counselling in general.

To access the online resources accompanying this chapter, please visit: https://study.sagepub.com/reevesandbond

2

What Is Counselling?

Chapter Overview

This chapter examines the wide range of uses of '**counselling**' in everyday life before looking at what counselling means as therapy and its distinguishing characteristics, particularly counsellors putting aside their own concerns and interests in order to hear and respond to clients' **issues**. An example of a definition designed to address international **diversity** is examined. The impact of official recognition and **regulation** is considered. This chapter concludes by discussing the relationship between counselling and other types of role – particularly as regards **psychotherapy, advice, guidance, befriending, advocacy, counselling skills** and **coaching**.

Key words

counselling, counseling, regulation, advice, advocacy, guidance, coaching, befriending, psychotherapy, counselling skills, **embedded counselling**

This book is about the use of '**counselling**' to promote the wellbeing of people who will often be seeking help at times of difficulty or vulnerability in their lives and the **ethics** that are needed to offer this type of help. However, the label 'counselling' is also used for many other types of activity and there is continued discussion within the field as to the differences and similarities between terms used, such as 'counselling', 'psychotherapy', 'therapy' and so on.

'Counselling' is a term that is used in many different ways. This explains why it carries such a wide range of meanings in everyday use. These include selling, as in 'double glazing counsellor'; advising, as in 'I counselled him to return to work as the longer he puts it off, the harder it will be'; or as in 'debt counselling', which can range from the fraudulent selling of unsuitable financial products to vulnerable people to highly professional and impartial help for financial difficulties.

There are also examples of the use of 'counselling' where the term has taken on a very narrow and technically specific meaning. 'Counselling', in some disciplinary proceedings, represents 'a serious talking to about the need to change behaviour', as a form of oral warning, which is the precursor of a written warning or dismissal. In this context, the interpersonal dynamics are both judgmental and authoritative. Counselling can also mean imparting expert **advice** in an authoritative manner, such as 'I counselled him to watch for problems with … but did he pay any attention?'

While these examples will be recognizable to most, the term 'counselling' has perhaps more recently been associated with mental health and a means of supporting people with emotional and relational distress. However, problems remain in that counselling can still mean different things to different people, at different times, and so the challenges of definition remain. Taking an international perspective is a good starting point, however.

The Meaning of 'Counselling' Internationally

At the international level there is a definite tendency to make the term 'counselling' all-encompassing in order to accommodate a **diversity** of cultures and practice. In languages where there is no equivalent to 'counselling', often the terms '**guidance**' or '**advice**' act as equivalents. Alternatively, the term 'counselling' is simply imported into the vocabulary of the language. The International Association for Counselling (IAC) has developed an all-encompassing definition that can be adapted to different national and social contexts. The tensions between being internationally inclusive and establishing a shared professional **identity** appear to be carefully balanced in this definition:

> The term 'counselling' has many meanings according to its cultural and professional context. Nonetheless it is possible to identify a definition that encompasses this diversity.

> Counselling may be described as a profession of relating and responding to others with the aim of providing them with opportunities to explore, clarify and work towards living in a more personally satisfying and resourceful way. Counselling may be applied to individuals, couples, families or groups and may be used in widely differing contexts and settings. (IAC, 2003: 6)

It is worth spending a few moments examining this definition carefully because it has been crafted to avoid being trapped within any therapeutic model or cultural context. The authors have stepped back from the characteristics of any particular practice or context to identify the key **issues** and features that are characteristic of counselling and indeed all types of talking or psychological therapies.

The activity is 'relating and responding to others', which not only covers all models of counselling but also the different styles of counselling adopted by different cultures, from authoritative advice based on careful listening and observation preferred in some traditional cultures to the most non-directive or facilitative styles of intervention favoured in some modern western cultures. Just as importantly it leaves open the question of whether the insight behind the style of intervention is based on following the ideas of a founding figure, philosophical **values** or **evidence-based practice**.

The purpose of counselling is 'to explore, clarify and work towards living in a more personally satisfying and resourceful way', which presents the work positively as being directed towards enhancing wellbeing rather than focusing on the negative experiences or difficulties that usually prompt someone to seek counselling. This increases the usefulness of the definition across cultures as mental **illness** and emotional difficulties usually carry some degree of stigma in most societies. However, the level of stigma is often much increased in cultures where avoiding 'shame' and 'loss of face' are paramount concerns for individuals and their families. In many traditional cultures in Asia and Africa, the mental illness of one person affects the reputation of all other family members in ways that physical illness may not. Employment and marriage prospects for all family members may be affected. Even moderate to serious mental illnesses may be experienced and communicated as aches and pains that are more easily accepted as physical illness rather than being viewed as a flaw in the character or personality of the person affected. For example, student health services often see a big difference in how international and home students in the UK react to the suggestion that they may be experiencing depression or anxiety. Home students generally accept the suggestion and want to engage in treatment plans. Some international students, particularly men from traditional cultures, will resist the thought of an emotional or psychological difficulty, stating a clear preference for a diagnosis of a physical illness that they see as far less damaging to their future prospects for marriage and employment or the reputation of their family. The focus on the positive purpose of counselling in this definition avoids inflaming resistance to counselling, even if it cannot totally resolve some cultural sensitivities about the emotional and psychological issues typically associated with counselling.

The IAC definition also leaves open the full range of possibilities for the types of issues that can be addressed by counselling. These might include empowering campaigners for **social justice**, enhancing performance in education and other settings, overcoming the effects of trauma or loss, mood management and improving relationships. The range of applications is unlimited. By placing the emphasis on positive improvement and wellbeing there is a strong message of hope which is psychologically so significant to improvement and recovery. This is a therapeutically sophisticated definition.

The last element of the definition emphasizes the potential variety of applications for counselling which include a wide range of clients, 'individuals, couples, families or groups'. There is also an explicit assertion of the adaptability and suitability of counselling for 'widely differing contexts and settings' (IAC, 2003: 6).

Even the spelling of 'counselling' varies between countries. The British English tradition is with a double 'll' whereas the US English preference is for a single 'l'. In many languages there is no verbal equivalent to counselling that can be used in translations. In these languages a translation of '**guidance**' or '**psychotherapy**' may be substituted, or the word 'counselling' may be imported into the language.

What is distinctive about this definition is its openness and positive embracing of difference between people and the applications of counselling. The majority of definitions incorporate position statements in favour of particular therapeutic models and/or specific services. It is appropriate to develop a definition that helps to inform potential users of that service about what to expect. This helps people to make informed choices and to shape expectations about using that service. More tightly defined approaches to counselling only become problematic if they claim to be the sole acceptable approach, and therefore aggravate rivalry and partisanship within what is a very creative field of professional activity that requires considerable flexibility in order to respond to different issues, client backgrounds and the settings in which counselling is delivered. The IAC definition is an example of a generic definition that has taken on the challenges of **cultural differences** and seems to be acceptable to an extremely wide range of different therapeutic approaches to and applications of counselling. The issues of **social diversity** will be frequently revisited throughout the book, but particularly in Chapter 12.

'Counselling' in the UK

There is long and varied use of 'counselling' in the UK, which predates the development of therapeutic counselling that ranges from giving **advice** 'betweene

Man to Man' (Bacon, 2008 [1625]) to a name for the criminal offence of counselling, that is, encouraging a crime in the Accessories and Abettors Act 1861. The term 'counselling' as a type of therapeutic and social intervention has its origins in the USA and was imported into the UK to address concerns about the impact of modern life on marriage and family life, leading to the creation of the Marriage Guidance Council in 1938 (now known as RELATE). CRUSE, the bereavement counselling service, started in 1959. The Central Advisory Council for Education (1963: section 233) envisaged the possibility of a full-time counsellor in large schools 'to be available to advise pupils throughout their school course and to prepare them for going out into the world', which prompted some of the first university courses in counselling.

Employee counselling services probably first started during the 1980s. The emergence of HIV/AIDS in the 1980s and 1990s provided another major stimulus for the development of psycho-social support, particularly during the early phase when the cause of the illness was unknown and effective treatments had yet to be developed. Even this incomplete and brief history reveals the range of applications to which counselling has been applied. This represents a considerable challenge for creating a definition that encompasses this diversity of practice and applications meaningfully.

The *Oxford English Dictionary* (2020) defines counselling as:

> The action of counsel v.; giving or taking of counsel; advising; spec. the giving of advice on personal, social, psychological, etc., problems as an occupation; in Psychology, a form of psychotherapy in which the counsellor adopts a permissive and supportive role in enabling a client to solve his or her own problems.

A definition prepared by the BACP during the protracted run-up to **regulation** of about twenty years captured the prevailing professional and ethical concerns about **privacy, confidentiality**, and protecting the **voluntary** nature of counselling:

> Counselling occurs when a counsellor sees a client in a private and confidential setting to explore a difficulty the client is having, distress they may be experiencing or perhaps their dissatisfaction with life or loss of a sense of direction and purpose. It is always at the request of the client and no one can properly be 'sent' for counselling. (BACP, 2008)

The Division of Counselling Psychology in the British Psychological Society (BPS) (2020) adopts a different definition to describe the careers and work undertaken by counselling psychologists:

> Counselling psychologists deal with a wide range of mental health problems concerning life issues including bereavement, domestic violence, sexual abuse, traumas and relationship issues. They understand diagnosis and the medical context to mental health problems and work with the individual's unique subjective psychological experience to empower their recovery and alleviate distress.

Counselling psychologists are a relatively new breed of professional applied psychologists concerned with the integration of psychological theory and research with therapeutic practice. The practice of counselling psychology requires a high level of self-awareness and competence in relating the skills and knowledge of personal and interpersonal dynamics to the therapeutic context.

A client's perspective may be significantly different from that of a counsellor:

> Clients want to be treated with respect, to be understood and helped to resolve problems … Clients want a counselling relationship that treats them as individuals and with hope. (Brainchild, 2008, cited in Aldridge, 2014: 17)

This client perspective is interesting as it is one of the very few that is the result of independent research commissioned by a professional body wanting to learn more about clients' perspectives than those of professionals. The specific mention of 'hope' reinforces the significance of a positive and forward-looking optimism that is focused on problem solving within a relationship founded on **respect** for them as people. In contemporary western **culture**, it is normal to think of ourselves as individuals first and then connected to others second. For the majority of the world population this would be the other way round. The primary **identity** is a collective identity connected to family (typically an extended family, clan or tribe) and any sense of individuality is secondary. This is explored more in Chapter 12.

If we examine the implications of these definitions for **ethical standards**, then some principles for practice emerge:

1. Counselling requires that a counsellor puts aside their own concerns and interests to focus attention on the client.
2. The goal is to address the issue, concern or problem that motivated the client to seek counselling.
3. The counsellor will be trained in order to undertake the role.
4. The methods used will vary according to the training, experience and knowledge of the counsellor, the characteristics of the client, and the setting.
5. Counselling usually takes place in a formal and agreed way between counsellor and client.

6. Professional ethics provide the basis for practice and public trust in a service that is usually provided at a time of personal distress or heightened vulnerability. The characteristic ethical challenges are avoiding the **exploitation** of clients in what may be an intimate emotional and psychological relationship with the counsellor and involve the **disclosure** of sensitive information about the client and others.

Counsellors are accountable to a combination of their clients, their professional body and/or their regulator who admitted them to a professional register for their ethics and standards, and especially the **safety** of clients. It is worth noting, however, that as the psychological therapies are not **statutorily regulated** in the UK (beyond 'counselling psychologist', which is regulated by the Health and Care Professions Council (HCPC) as part of the **practitioner psychologist** titles), a counsellor is not required to be a member of a professional body and thus may not be subject to any regulatory control. Counsellors who are not members of a professional body may act independently of any ethical framework or guidance and, in turn, not be accountable for their professional conduct. Much work has been undertaken by the key professional bodies in the UK that represent the psychological therapies to offer public education to ensure that clients go to counsellors who hold a professional association membership, are listed on a register and therefore are accountable for their actions; that is, the client has the right to recourse to a complaints process should the need arise. The establishment of a voluntary register, accredited by the Professional Standards Authority (PSA), has been an important development in this area. As this is a system of accredited voluntary registration, there is no restriction on who may call themselves counsellors or offer services as counsellors, but it is only those on the register who may call themselves 'registered counsellors' and promote their services using the register's logo. The PSA is promoting this scheme to the public as the best way of selecting a practitioner through the directory of accredited voluntary registers with confidence.

The primary purpose of both systems of regulation is the protection of the public by providing an easy way of checking who is registered and has met the required standards. There are also disciplinary processes by which members of the public can raise concerns about particular practitioners and their fitness to practise. If these concerns are considered serious enough to require a hearing in which the case against the practitioner is proven, this may lead to the person concerned being struck off the register or less serious sanctions. The outcome that appears to worry practitioners the most is having a judgment against them posted on the official website with details of the hearing for all to see. Current cases and recent judgments can usually be found on the websites of the registering bodies.

Voluntary Registration and Future Developments

The introduction of the PSA register for counselling and psychotherapy has arguably been an important step forward in providing important safeguards for clients accessing therapy, supporting the development of professional conduct processes to hold to account poor or harmful practice, and for professional bodies to clearly articulate counselling in a way to build public confidence. At the time of writing there are 11 counselling and psychotherapy PSA accredited registers in the UK:

- Association of Child Psychotherapists (ACP)
- Association of Christian Counsellors (ACC)
- British Association for Counselling and Psychotherapy (BACP)
- British Association of Play Therapists
- British Psychoanalytic Council (BPC)
- COSCA (Counselling and Psychotherapy in Scotland)
- Human Givens Institute (HGI)
- National Counselling Society (NCS)
- National Hypnotherapy Society
- UK Association for Humanistic Psychology Practitioners (UKAHPP)
- UK Council for Psychotherapy (UKCP)

It is difficult to provide a full account of membership across these organizations, as each one has a different approach to publishing membership figures. A formal collaboration was formed between three of the register holders: BACP, BPC and UKCP, which began in earnest around 2015–2016. While each organization retained full independence from the others, the collaboration facilitated areas for joint work across practice development, professional standards and advocacy for the profession, and was led by the respective Chairs, CEOs and operational teams. The approximate membership total for these three organizations is around 70,000, giving some insight into the extent of registrants across all 11 PSA registers.

This collaboration in many ways was a step towards greater coherence in the profession, allowing key bodies to make representations to stakeholders, commissioners and politicians whereas before the profession had been accused of having a fractured voice. However, this early work has the potential for wider collaboration in the future involving other register holders. A shared aim for the profession is for it to speak with a more united voice, albeit the detail of that voice is still to be determined.

Social Justice in Context

The PSA register and emerging collaborative relationships also have the potential to put in mechanism to respond to the ever-potential for the statutory regulation of the profession. There are strong arguments for and against statutory regulation, some arguing that it will provide meaningful safeguards for clients; offer status and legitimacy long-awaited for the profession; support the development of national pay scales; and continue to support best practice in training. Those opposing statutory regulation argue that no greater client protection will be achieved than is already available through a voluntary process; that the unique contribution counselling and psychotherapy have to offer those experiencing mental health distress will be undermined; that statutory regulation can often miss important nuances in professions and deliver a framework that 'misses the point'; and that state regulation has no place philosophically in the delivery of therapy. The arguments for and against are often heated and impassioned, and no clear united view has emerged.

The current position held by UK governments has been against statutory regulation and rather for the active support of the voluntary, PSA-managed process. The importance of public protection has, however, always trumped other issues and some believe a major public protection concern coming to light might quickly change the landscape and government position. Greater working collaboration between professional associations and the PSA perhaps position the profession such that, should the day come, the profession will be better placed to respond to those challenges than when statutory regulation was last mooted.

Pause for Reflection

Consider your own training or practice as a counsellor and your experience of voluntary regulation. What are your views about the relative benefits and costs of statutory regulation, and what informs your position?

Counselling and Other Roles

There are many different ways of providing assistance to people by listening and talking. Each requires certain types of expertise and ways of supporting the client effectively. For members of the public, understanding the differences between roles may help them find the most appropriate help. For counsellors, understanding the differences may help them point clients towards the most suitable services or recognize when they are combining roles within their counselling and consider the ethical implications of doing this. In the more recent developments of their Ethical Framework, the BACP adopted the term '**counselling professions**' to be more inclusive of a range of associated activities, such as **counselling**, **psychotherapy**, **counselling skills** and **coaching**. These, and others, are explored more here.

Advice

Advice is an opinion given to someone about what would be the best action to take. It usually entails giving a person information about the choices open to them and then, from a position of greater expertise or authority, a recommendation as to the best course of action. Rosalind Brooke (1972), writing about Citizens Advice Bureaux, describes the advisory process as having two aspects: 'The advisor not only may interpret the information in order to sort it to the needs of the enquirer, but may also offer an opinion about the wisdom of obtaining a solution in a particular way.' Giving advice requires expert knowledge about the subject that is causing the client concern in order to identify potential solutions or the best way forward. The best advisers will present options and have the skills to help clients choose between them. This description highlights the difficulty that 'advice' poses for counsellors.

The aim of counselling is to enable clients to discover their own wisdom rather than have wisdom imparted to them by counsellors. The counselling process is intended to increase the client's ability to take control rather than depend on another. This difference between counselling and advice does not mean that advice is an inappropriate way of offering help. It is a different method and perhaps more suitable for practical problems than for making decisions about relationships, or coping with transitions or other psychosocial issues. Advice is particularly suitable for legal and financial issues or for understanding how administrative or technological systems work and getting the best out of them.

Recent developments in **evidence-based practice** for the talking therapies means that the knowledge base behind counselling on issues like recovering from depression or managing anxiety is growing, and that sometimes it is appropriate to share that information with clients and help them apply it to their own situation. However, when advice is incorporated within counselling it is usually provided within a way of working that is directed at improving client expertise and their control over the issues concerning them.

Guidance

Guidance has been used in as many different ways as 'counselling'. During the late 1960s and the 1970s (a time when guidance services were expanding rapidly in social welfare and education) the terms 'guidance' and 'counselling' could be used interchangeably.

It appears that some time since the 1970s the use of 'guidance' has developed in two different directions. One trend has emphasized the kinds of values and methods of working associated with counselling. This trend is characterized by a very strong emphasis on working in ways that enable recipients of guidance to make their own decisions. In this sense the guide is like a signpost, pointing out different possible routes and helping people to select their own destinations and ways of getting there. Information-giving and advising may be more prominent in workers' interventions than would be the case in counselling, but the emphasis on values based on client **autonomy** mean that this form of guidance is very closely related to counselling and, in some instances, these are the same kind of activity. This use of 'guidance' has become well established in educational settings and is encouraged by many writers and commentators on educational advice, guidance and counselling services (Ali and Graham, 1996; Gothard et al., 2001; Evans, 2009).

An alternative use of 'guidance' that appears from time to time is to offer guidance in a more authoritative way that relies on the expertise of the source of guidance to indicate the benefits of following that guidance and the adverse consequences of failing to do so. In health campaigns 'counselling' has been used to signal patient-led decisions on matters such as whether to be tested for particular health conditions, where the outcome of the tests may be psychologically challenging and the balance of benefits and harm therefore uncertain or unknown in the current state of knowledge. 'Counselling' in this health context is closest to an extended discussion about informed consent or the refusal of a particular service or treatment. 'Guidance' is offered as a more authoritative intervention when the medical knowledge is well established and the consequences of failing to act on it may have serious consequences for the patient. Guidance in this sense has been used effectively in reducing smoking and excessive alcohol consumption. Cardiovascular, diabetes and sexual health clinics frequently incorporate guidance within the services they offer.

The distinctive feature of guidance is the professional's commitment to moving someone along a path from a current state to a more desired state. In the less directive approaches to guidance a client's views will be supported and engaged with. In more authoritative guidance, the guide may emphasize and explain the benefits of following the guidance. Resistance to well-informed but unwelcome guidance may act as an effective psychological defence for an extended period of time. However, if that defence collapses, the person concerned may require psychological support around underlying issues that may be best met by counselling.

Advocacy

Whether or not **advocacy** has a place in the delivery of therapy is debated by some: on one hand it is viewed as an overly political position that has no philosophical fit with offering support for mental health distress; on the other it is argued that if therapy is, in part, helping clients to find a voice, advocacy is a critically important part of that process. At a simple level 'advocacy', its usage dating back in language to ~1520, might be defined as 'to support, recommend or speak in favour of' (OED, 2020); its Latin origins, from *advocatia*, means to 'summon, call to one's aid'. In the context of the counselling professions, it might mean supporting a client, a couple or group, to argue for their position or for change, often in a **social justice** sense.

Dalrymple and Boylan (2013: 3) offer two primary types of advocacy in a social work context:

1. *Case- or issue-based advocacy*, where work is focused with individuals or small groups such as families in a task-centred way.
2. *Systemic or cause advocacy*, where knowledge from individual cases contributes to collective advocacy for systemic change to legislation, policy or practice.

It is possible to consider both these types of advocacy within the context of the counselling professions. Counsellors in college or university settings, for example, might regularly write a letter or email of support for a student attending as a client who has missed coursework due to mental health distress, or whose attendance at university is being considered. This would be an example of case- or issue-based advocacy. However, that same counsellor working in an education setting might see a number of students over the course of an academic year with similar presenting problems apparently exacerbated by a particular department, where procedures or actions taken by the department might have led to particular difficulties. The counsellor, or counselling service, raising these concerns with the institution for consideration might be an example of systemic or cause advocacy.

There is a growing movement that positions the counselling professions within a political frame, in that mental health is inextricably linked to social factors (in addition to other factors too), that some assert it is impossible to separate out one from the other. Several professional associations have embedded social justice as a central aspect of their strategy (e.g. BACP). By doing so, a recognition is made as to the importance of social, political, cultural and environmental factors in the work of a professional association and how strategy is located accordingly. Some groups have actively argued this position for many years, such as Psychotherapists and Counsellors for Social Responsibility (PCSR). With that perspective, an advocacy role – either for individual clients, or the advocacy of systemic change – becomes a given rather than an optional 'bolt-on'.

Befriending and listening

The best known of organizations committed to providing a listening service is the Samaritans. The use of **befriending** to counter the social isolation of specific groups of people is a goal shared by all providers of this type of service. Their social isolation may be due to physical circumstances (e.g. people who are housebound due to illness or **disability**), or public attitudes (e.g. people who are mentally ill or have learning difficulties, the dying, and offenders). The current isolation of increasing numbers of elderly people living alone is a growing social crisis which is particularly suited to befriending services such as those developed by Age UK and other similar organizations.

Counsellors and befrienders share common values about the importance of listening and doing so in a non-judgmental way, but the way they construct that relationship will be different. Counsellors tend to work within a formal **contract** with **boundaries** both in the contacts between practitioner and client and in the types of service being offered. In contrast, befrienders may be more flexible regarding boundaries in relationships by meeting other people in a client's life or introducing them to their own friends or family. They may have meals together, visit a pub or cafe, or go for a walk or to the cinema. Personal **disclosure** by the befriender may also be as free and as unconstrained as would be the case with friendship. Befriending may not be confined to talking and listening in the way it often is in counselling. A befriender may also offer practical help, such as accompanying someone to the shops or even getting their shopping, and helping with cooking or gardening.

Counselling and psychotherapy

For many years the BACP held that it is not possible to make a generally accepted distinction between **counselling** and **psychotherapy**. In this respect, it followed well-founded traditions which use the terms interchangeably in contrast to others that distinguish them. Latterly, however, in the context of collaborative work with UKCP and BPC, and in the form of a project focusing on training standards and practice requirements for counselling and psychotherapy (SCoPEd), BACP shifted from this long-held position and began to argue a differentiation, based on training entry routes and practice, between 'counselling' and 'psychotherapy'. While this garnered some support, the initial proposal document was received with anger and hostility by some members who believed an epistemological fracture had occurred in the perceived introduction of a hierarchy of helping, with counselling subsequently devalued in favour of psychotherapy. The collaboration of BACP, UKCP and BPC argued this was not the intention, but acknowledged major flaws in the initial consultation document. At the time of writing, a second iteration of the **SCoPEd** framework was released for further consultation (SCoPEd, 2020b). This will be discussed further in Chapter 8.

When the terms 'counselling' and 'psychotherapy' are used in their widest sense they are the same. On the other hand, these terms are sometimes used to distinguish between two roles. The historical origins of psychotherapy are closely related to attempts to find ways of curing mental illness, especially in the USA (McLeod, 1998). The direct influence of psychoanalytic ideas is more evident in psychotherapy than in counselling. As a consequence, some people have sought to establish clear distinctions between counselling and psychotherapy on the assumption that responding to mental health issues requires working at a greater depth (see Table 2.1).

TABLE 2.1 *The characteristics of counselling and psychotherapy (adapted from Brammer and Shostrum, 1982)*

Counselling characteristics	Psychotherapy characteristics
Educational	Reconstructive
Situational	Issues arising from personality
Problem solving	Analytic
Conscious awareness	Pre-conscious and unconscious
Emphasis on working with people who do not have severe or persistent emotional problems	Emphasis on 'neurotics' or working with persistent and/or severe emotional problems
Focus on the present	Focus on the past
Shorter length of contract	Longer length of contract

Attempts to distinguish counselling and psychotherapy have proved problematic in the UK. Many people with a psychodynamic background would tend to support the existence of a distinction linked to the history of this approach and a much stronger sense of professional hierarchy through psychodynamic counselling, psychotherapy and psychoanalysis. Entitlement to progress through the hierarchy and to work in greater depth with clients is linked to levels of training and personal therapy or analysis, as outlined in the SCoPEd (2020b) framework document. Some humanistic approaches to therapy have adopted similarly structured professional hierarchies, such as transactional analysis. These hierarchical approaches to different levels of therapy position counselling as dealing with problems that are primarily pressures from the outside environment, rather than deeply embedded difficulties resulting in rigid neurotic patterns.

In this hierarchical approach, counselling is restricted to helping people who have the capacity to cope in most circumstances but who are experiencing temporary difficulties, or making transitions or adjustments in their life. Issues arising from difficult relationships at home, making decisions, coping with serious illness, bereavement, addiction and so on may all be within the scope of counselling. If issues are merely symptomatic of something deeper, or the client is experiencing more entrenched problems such as persistent phobias, anxiety states, low self-esteem or difficulty in establishing relationships, then psychotherapy may be more appropriate. This would imply the need for a difference in training and expertise between counsellors and psychotherapists. This position would additionally support an argument of the importance of viewing clients in their systemic frame: their political, social, cultural and demographic profile and how their experience of distress and subsequent presentation in counselling had been shaped by factors outside of their control.

In a paper delivered to the 16th Annual Training Conference of the British Association for Counselling (BAC), Brian Thorne (1992) suggested that the quest for difference between counselling and psychotherapy was illogical and invalid. He argued that implicit in the kinds of distinctions most frequently made between counselling and psychotherapy was the idea that counselling was concerned with cognitive problems and psychotherapy with affective problems. He debunked this line of argument in the following way:

> I would suggest that it takes only a moment's reflection to reveal the uselessness of such distinctions. Clearly, cognition and affect are both involved in all behaviours. No choice, for example, can ever be simply logical and rational. What is more, a serious personality problem usually brings with it many situational and environmental dilemmas and a situational problem may well have its source in a personality disturbance. It would, of course, be highly convenient if problems could be categorised and circumscribed so neatly but to suggest that they can is to fly in the face of the facts.

In his paper he argues against all the distinctions between counselling and psychotherapy made by Brammer and Shostrum (1982) and many others. There is no doubt that this debate will continue for some considerable time, further fuelled perhaps by the SCoPEd consultation, and that ultimately it may have more to do with status and money than with substantive differences. Some suggest that in private practice the label 'psychotherapy' attracts higher fees from clients than 'counselling'. However, there is a great deal of common ground between counselling and psychotherapy. Clients talk about their experience of being on the receiving end of counselling or psychotherapy in very similar terms. Fee differentials notwithstanding, the difference between the two appears to be more important to practitioners than to clients.

From an ethical perspective, it is clear that counsellors and psychotherapists work within the same ethical framework. It may be that if differences between the two roles can be established, there will be some corresponding differences in **standards** of practice or training, but even these may simply be details in comparison to the many standards shared in common.

Pause for Reflection

Consider your work as a 'therapist' and the training you undertook, or are undertaking, to reach that point. Would you consider your work to be that of a 'counsellor', a 'psychotherapist', or is there another descriptor that suits your work better? What factors inform your thinking and to what extent do you consider the use of terms to be about status or accuracy?

Counselling skills and embedded counselling

The development of a distinction between **counselling** and **counselling skills** has played a significant part in enabling the development of counselling as a distinct professional role. However, the notion of counselling skills remains controversial and is much criticized by those who prefer **embedded counselling.** This section will set out how 'counselling skills' emerged as a term for particular types of activity before considering the criticisms of this development. Although there were early advocates for 'counselling skills' (Bond, 1989), it is important to recognize that there is some validity in the concerns about this development. This review will begin by considering a common misunderstanding.

The most obvious misunderstanding is based on the idea that 'counselling skills' is a label for a set of activities unique to counselling. Although the term is sometimes used in this way, it is quickly discredited because any attempt to list specific 'counselling skills' (e.g. active listening, paraphrasing, using open questions, reflective responses etc.) immediately looks indistinguishable from lists labelled 'social skills', 'communication skills', 'interpersonal skills' and so on. In order to understand what is meant by 'counselling skills', it is useful to take the two words separately (McLeod and McLeod, 2011; Reeves, 2018).

'Counselling' is an indication of the source of the concept historically. It shows that even though these skills are not unique to counselling, it is the way they have been articulated in counselling that has been useful to other roles. For example, advice-giving has a much longer history than counselling skills, but the tendency has been to concentrate on the content of the advice rather than the way it is delivered. However, the methods advisers use to communicate with clients can be adapted to improve the way advice is given and maximize client involvement in the decision making. 'Counselling' in this context is acknowledging the source of the concept and method of communication. Similarly, nurses, tutors, personnel managers, social workers and many others have all recognized that there are advantages in adapting the methods of communication used in counselling to aspects of their own role. One way in which an outside observer might detect that counselling skills are being used is by the pattern of communication. This is illustrated in Table 2.2.

TABLE 2.2 *Differences in communication*

Style	Pattern of flow	Time ratio
Imparting expertise	Interactor → Recipient	80:20
Conversation	Interactor → Recipient	50:50
Counselling skills	Interactor → Recipient	20:80

When counselling skills are being used, an outside observer might notice that the recipient is encouraged to take greater control of the dialogue's agenda than in other styles of communication. The values implicit in the use of counselling skills are similar to those for counselling which place an emphasis on a client's capacity for self-determination in how help is sought as well as for any decisions or actions that may result.

The term 'skills' in 'counselling skills' is sometimes taken in a very literal sense to mean 'discrete behaviours', but this is not the way the term is understood in the social sciences. Skills that are used to enhance relationships can be distinguished from 'physical skills' (as in sport or work) and 'mental' and 'intellectual' skills, not merely on the basis of observable behaviours. These are inextricably linked to the goal of the person using them. For instance, Michael Argyle (1981) states that 'by socially skilled behaviour I mean behaviour which is effective in realising the goals of the interactor'. In the context of counselling skills, those goals are to implement the values of counselling by assisting the self-expression and autonomy of the recipient.

One of the ways in which an independent observer might be able to distinguish between 'counselling skills' and 'counselling' is whether the contract is explicit between the two people. This is highlighted in one of the alternative definitions of counselling which is still in popular use: 'People become engaged in counselling when a person, occupying regularly or temporarily the role of counsellor, offers or agrees explicitly to offer time, attention or respect to another person or persons temporarily in the role of client' (BAC, 1984). This definition was originally devised to distinguish between spontaneous or *ad hoc* counselling and formal counselling. The overt nature of the latter, involving 'offers' and explicit agreements, was seen as 'the dividing line between the counselling task and the *ad hoc* counselling and is the major safeguard of the rights of the consumer' (BAC, 1985). This definition also provides a useful basis for distinguishing when someone is using counselling skills in a role other than that of counsellor or when they are counselling.

This set of views provides the basis for determining when counselling skills are being used:

- when there is intentional use of specific interpersonal skills which reflect the values of counselling;
- when the practitioner's primary role (e.g. nurse, tutor, line manager, social worker, personnel officer, helper) is enhanced without being changed;
- when the client perceives the practitioner as acting within their primary professional or caring role which is not that of being a counsellor.

The values of counselling would focus on respecting a client's values, experience, thoughts, feelings and their capacity for self-determination, and aiming to serve the best interests of that client.

There are three frequent misconceptions often encountered in discussions about counselling skills:

1. *Using counselling skills is always a lower-order activity than counselling*: This is not the case. Arguably, the user of counselling skills may be working under more demanding circumstances than the counsellor, who usually has the benefit of more extended periods of time which have already been agreed in advance. In comparison, the user of counselling skills may be working more opportunistically with much less certainty about the duration of the encounter. Users of counselling skills can be more or less skilled, just like counsellors. However, using counselling skills is not a role in itself but to enhance the performance of another role. This means that the capacity to use counselling skills effectively depends not only on being skilled in their use but also on someone's **competence** in their primary role (e.g. a nurse, a tutor). For all these reasons, some people may require a higher level of competence to use counselling skills than may be required in counselling. It certainly cannot be assumed that using counselling skills is a lower level of activity.
2. *People in occupational roles, other than counsellor, cannot counsel*: This would mean that doctors, nurses, youth workers and so on cannot counsel but can only use counselling skills. This is not the case. With appropriate training, counselling supervision and clear contracting with the client in ways consistent with counselling, it seems that anyone can change to take on the role of 'counsellor'.

There are key issues about keeping the boundaries between different roles clear and managing overlapping roles or dual relationships, but not all dual relationships are undesirable provided the boundary between the relationships can be clearly identified and is respected by both counsellor and client. Usually it is easier, whenever possible, to avoid the potential pitfalls of dual relationships by ensuring that a counsellor is independent of the provision of other services and other relationships, whether personal or professional, to a client.

3. *Anyone with the occupational title 'counsellor' is always counselling*: This is not the case. As the concept of counselling has narrowed down into a specifically contracted role, there is a need for 'counsellors' to distinguish between when they are counselling and when they are performing other roles, such as training, supervision, managing or advocacy. In each of these other roles a counsellor is likely to be using counselling skills.

The distinction between counselling skills and counselling may have been helpful in pursuing the professionalization of counselling as a distinct role, by distinguishing a more defined approach to counselling from situations where someone uses a more loosely defined approach to using counselling to support some other helping role (such as being a tutor, a health worker or another role that has its own identity and expertise). Professionally, within organizations like the BACP, the creation of counselling skills has provided the conceptual and political space to give better focused attention to what is entailed ethically to being a counsellor. The complications of other professional cultures and constraints could then be set aside in order to concentrate on counselling as it was developing, in all its variations, as a specialized service. Such distinctions can lead to unequal attention being given to each part so that one becomes favoured over another, and in this case one type of role (i.e. counselling) becomes more central to professional development than the other. This fragmenting of roles can have undesirable consequences. The process of defining and restricting professional identity, even if it is to advance ethical and professional standards, cannot avoid problems associated with becoming more exclusive and professionally inward-looking.

The idea of the **embedded counsellor** provides a substantial challenge to such exclusivity and may prove to be a useful remedy to any exaggerated sense of professional identity by redirecting attention to the extent to which counselling is used in its wider sense within so many other types of helping role and reaffirming the value of such work. McLeod and McLeod (2011) have written eloquently in favour of the embedded counsellor. They argue that it is socially and culturally important to explicitly acknowledge all the counselling that takes place in brief episodes embedded within other professional tasks (e.g. teaching, nursing and career advice).

The concept of the 'embedded counsellor' is a welcome development if it helps to rebuild links with other professions that may have been broken in the quest for a professional identity for counsellors and revives a shared focus on the humanizing values that are so precious in everyday living. Approached in this way, the use of the label 'embedded counsellor' invites us to re-engage with the radical values that prompted the origins of counselling in ways that are relevant to current life.

Regardless of whether 'counselling skills' or 'embedded counselling' is the preferred terminology, this type of emotionally intelligent engagement with people in challenging circumstances by teachers, nurses, social workers and many other professions is highly desirable, and may often be the difference between being effective or ineffective.

Coaching

Coaching is in its unregulated phase of creative formation with many different positions and claims to professional territory. Coaching is directed towards the improvement of performance by skilled tutoring within a designated area of life. The word 'tutoring' rather than 'teaching' is used here because the best coaches arguably not only draw on their own expertise but also facilitate the learning of the person being coached (sometimes referred to as a 'coachee'). Rogers (2012: 7) defines coaching as:

> a partnership of equals whose aim is to achieve speedy, increased and sustainable effectiveness through focused learning in every aspect of the client's life. Coaching raises self-awareness and identifies choices.

'Executive coaches' tutor managers in the art of leadership and may have specialist knowledge about leadership in particular types of organizations. 'Sports coaches' work on the technical skills, strategy and psychology required to succeed in particular sports. 'Life coaching' is probably closest to counselling but is often directed towards specific issues.

Coaching is characteristically future-looking and striving for improvement by developing strategies and skills for success. It tends to be time-limited, requires the coach to be skilled in the issues under consideration, and to be able to evaluate and give feedback on performance. Personal issues may be discussed but the primary focus is on that performance. This is probably the critical difference between coaching and counselling. In coaching the focus is on an issue selected by the client as something they would like to perform better: 'How can I prepare better for a job interview?', 'How can I improve my feedback-giving skills?',

'How can I relate better to my colleagues?' It is usually also future-looking. Counselling often starts with a less specific focus to address a more general problem, such as an emotional difficulty, problems in relationships, trauma or difficult transitions. The work is often about addressing broader issues in greater depth in order to resolve some form of personal or psychological difficulty. In counselling, someone's past may feature more than in coaching.

A great deal of thought has been given within the BACP about the compatibility between counselling and coaching. The first chair of the Coaching Division observed that:

> there are many skillful, ethical and highly trained coaches (with and without a therapeutic background), who do life enhancing work with clients right across the spectrum – including coaching youngsters to help them overcome being bullied, coaching ex-offenders to develop confidence and avoid reoffending, working with organisations to help them to lead and manage people fairly, effectively and with integrity, and helping 'ordinary' people to find and fulfil their potential.

Since that time, the Coaching Division of BACP has flourished and is seen as an integral part of the work of the Association. Their most recent stated strategy talks of the development of coaching competencies, a Certificate of Proficiency and subsequent coaching register as well as the development of good practice guidelines (BACP: Coaching, 2020a).

Mentoring

Mentoring is a supportive relationship designed to assist someone with difficult transitions, compensate for disadvantages in their life, or sustain challenging roles. A mentor will usually have relevant experience in overcoming the issues faced by a mentee and therefore can provide inspiration as a role model and also provide well-informed advice, coaching or embedded counselling.

Mentoring is widely used in some settings to support people through the transition into a new role or across life stages where a more experienced and established person offers their support to someone less secure or experienced. It can be used to support motivation and help to lift aspirations, particularly those of young people and especially of those who may be moving into unfamiliar environments or professional cultures. Mentoring has been used with looked-after children as compensation for the lack of family support. Like coaching, there is a strong focus on learning through discussion and dialogue.

Mentoring is widely used in professional contexts to support people taking on new professional roles or posts. These relationships are usually for specific purposes or defined periods of time. Counselling supervision is arguably a form of professional mentoring designed to ensure the sustainability of working with emotionally and relationally challenging issues. The full range of purposes for this application of mentoring is considered in Chapter 14. What makes this unusual is that it is sustained across the working life of counsellors as an ethical requirement. Registrants of the BACP-accredited voluntary register have to be prepared to be audited about their use of supervision. This demonstrates that this version of mentoring combines support with **accountability**. As with all the other roles considered, there is considerable versatility in how these are applied.

The Emergence of the Counselling Professions

The above discussion of the activities related to 'counselling' demonstrates the shades of grey that sit across how they are defined. That is, while there are clear similarities, as have been outlined, there are many differences too and finding discrete aspects to differentiate them is sometimes notoriously difficult. This isn't simply an academic challenge either: as professional associations work to strengthen and develop their good practice and ethical guidance to members, they need to attend carefully to the profile of their member activities to ensure that guidance is inclusive and representative of their diverse cohort, rather than too narrowly defined, thus missing some of what is being offered to clients.

The *Ethical Framework for Good Practice in Counselling and Psychotherapy* (2013) was re-written and launched by BACP in 2016 under the re-titled *Ethical Framework for the Counselling Professions*, later updated in 2018 (BACP, 2018a). Led by Professor Tim Bond, this re-drafting of the core ethical guidance all members signed up to was a undertaking and represented an important shift with a more inclusive title. Aspects of the *Ethical Framework* were heavily consulted on, including the use of the term 'counselling professions' as opposed to 'counselling and psychotherapy'. There was very little dissent for this change and a great deal more support. This perhaps spoke of the diversity of practice amongst the Association's membership and affirmed the value of the change in title.

The current *Ethical Framework* defines 'counselling professions' as providers of services informed by therapeutic theory and practice that are delivered with sufficient expertise to satisfy professional standards and ethics. These professions include coaching, counselling, pastoral care, psychotherapy and using counselling skills (BACP, 2018a). With that in mind, therefore, it is our intention to use the term 'counselling professions' throughout this text in considering the standards and ethics that apply to activities in an inclusive way, other than when there is a need to make a clear distinction between them.

Conclusion

One of the characteristics of a modern industrial and technologically based society is the creation of specialized roles to address specific tasks. The boundaries between these roles can be fiercely defended by professionals who have invested time and money in training and gaining the appropriate expertise and therefore understandably want to protect their livelihoods. However, these roles evolve and change over time and may be completely overtaken by developments in new technology. As can be seen in this chapter, roles that rely on listening and talking to assist with personal and social problems are indeed still evolving and the boundaries between them are altering over time.

This makes it difficult to define different roles permanently or to be too adamant about which role is most suitable for which type of issue. There are considerable variations in how each role can be applied. With these cautions about not being too rigid in how the definitions are applied, it is possible to have working definitions that can distinguish such roles and the issues for which they are particularly suitable.

Table 2.3 offers a short statement about the distinctive characteristics and examples of the sorts of issues for which each role is particularly suitable. Because the definitions are so problematic and the role boundaries are disputed, the table should be regarded as offering a suggested position and a starting point from which to consider how to view the differences between roles and their applications.

TABLE 2.3 *Role characteristics and applications*

Role	Characteristics	Examples of typical applications
Counselling/ psychotherapy	Based on attentive listening and focused interventions to help someone overcome a significant difficulty in their lives	Emotional difficulties Relationship difficulties Mild to moderate mental illness Recovery from trauma or loss
Befriending	Provides social and personal support by offering companionship and practical help	Social isolation Challenging personal circumstances due to illness, disability or social prejudice

(Continued)

TABLE 2.3 *(Continued)*

Role	Characteristics	Examples of typical applications
Advising	Provides an informed opinion about how best to achieve what the inquirer is seeking	Used whenever specialized knowledge about the issues in question is required – particularly useful for technical, procedural or administrative issues
Guiding/offering guidance	Similar to advising but on issues requiring more extended consideration or involving more significant issues for the inquirer	Careers guidance Health guidance Changing lifestyle
Using counselling skills/ embedded counselling	Provides ways of responding constructively to the emotions of people receiving education, health or social care, or other professional services	Supporting someone in an emotionally challenging situation Problem solving
Coaching	Supporting someone to overcome a challenging task or enhance the performance of particular skills	Preparation in advance of a competitive event such as a job interview or assessment Enhancing existing skills or performance in the workplace
Mentoring	Building capability and providing support over major personal transitions	People negotiating major changes in their lives, especially if their circumstances lack some of the support available to others in similar situations Passing hard-won learning and experience to successors in developing their wisdom

What is counselling?

Eight people talk about an issue they are facing and the sort of help they would like. What sort of help do you think would be most suitable?

'Counselling' is used in this book to refer to a role and type of activity delivered in accordance with professional standards that emphasize the ethical significance of enabling clients to increase their capacity to act for themselves and gain an improved sense of personal wellbeing. This means that there will be times when counsellors must work in ways that will overlap with or draw upon expertise learnt in other roles. There may also be times when a client's needs may be better met by referral to a different type of service. With so many closely related roles and the considerable variability in their availability to particular clients, counsellors will need to continue to be creative in how they develop their own roles and relate to the other roles considered in this chapter. However, it is also important to acknowledge that each of these roles has a distinctive tradition and associated areas of expertise. With the relevant expertise and professional support, it may be possible to incorporate aspects of these successfully within counselling to meet specific client needs, particularly when referral is not a viable option. Nonetheless counselling ethics and standards would apply.

To access the online resources accompanying this chapter, please visit: https://study.sagepub.com/reevesandbond

3

Sources of Counselling Ethics

Chapter Overview

This chapter examines six potential sources of **ethics** for working with clients and their application in **counselling**.

Key words

personal ethics, therapeutic **values, agency policy, codes**, frameworks, ethical **guidance**, moral philosophy, **law**

The construction of **counselling ethics** is fundamentally a social process which draws upon many different sources of ethical insight. Often these sources agree on what is the right or best way to act, but this is not always the case. Differences between current concerns and contexts may lead to different views. Careful consideration of any divergences in ethical direction is usually the best way forward in developing an ethical position. Each of the sources can be regarded as a different kind of ethical narrative which requires careful consideration to test how well it fits the situation facing counsellor and client.

It is important for counsellors to ask questions of themselves to enable them to identify ethical issues or dilemmas that emerge in their practice, and how they have navigated them. Often counsellors generally draw upon a selection of six sources:

1. Personal ethics
2. Ethics implicit in therapeutic models
3. Agency policy
4. Professional **codes**, frameworks and guidelines
5. Moral philosophy
6. Law

The urgency of a situation may restrict the choice to one or two sources and greater reflection may expand the choice beyond six. In these circumstances, presenting six sources rather than any other number is somewhat arbitrary. The list could easily have been expanded to include religious and political sources or contracted to exclude moral philosophy. A rationale for excluding the former two is the sense that the direct influence of any religious and political source tends to be downplayed by counsellors in the interests of respecting their clients' **values**. As a consequence, religious and political beliefs tend to be included within a counsellor's personal ethics and values; conversely, including moral philosophy is based on ethical discussions involving counsellors. It is apparent that when ideas derived from moral philosophy have been mentioned, these are valued as a source of language and concepts for examining ethical issues. It would be difficult to have a credible professional ethic that did not take into account insights derived from moral philosophy. The six ethical sources of counselling ethics are represented in Figure 3.1.

Personal Ethics

Taking on a professional role may create a tension between personal ethics and those you would consider appropriate to your role. This is most evident if you think about how you would respond to a friend or a client in similar circumstances. What may seem ethical in one relationship may seem inappropriate in the other.

One clear example comes to mind. A counsellor who learnt that a friend was considering dating someone with a serious infectious **illness** considered how he had discovered that information. If he had learnt about the risk of infection from a social conversation, he would feel entitled to warn his friend. On the other hand, if he had discovered it from his work, he would feel obliged to remain silent. This dichotomy of ethical responses can be very uncomfortable and raise fundamental choices between personal and professional integrity. However, the degree of separation

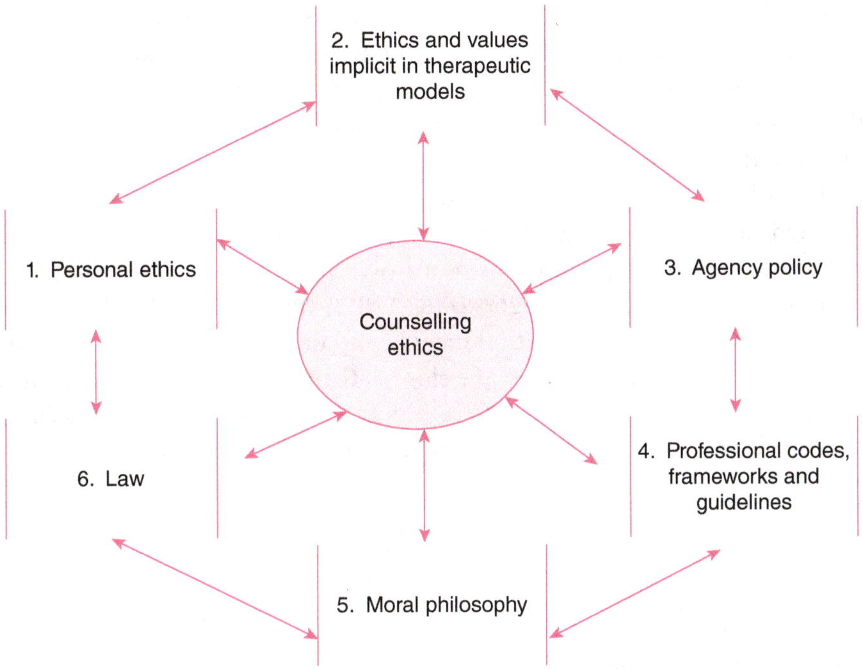

FIGURE 3.1 *Sources of professional ethics*

between personal and professional ethics is probably an inevitable part of adapting to a specialized role and taking into account the collective ethic of other members of that profession.

Pause for Reflection

Consider the scenario above: do you agree that the two situations might lead to different conclusions? If not, why, and if so what factors would inform your perspective?

Counsellors who seem most at ease with this dichotomy appear to recognize a distinction between their personal and professional ethic but have integrated *both* ethics within a deeper sense of self. As a consequence, a potentially contradictory dichotomy is more likely to be experienced as complementary aspects of the same person, whether that person is viewing themself from the inside or is viewed from the outside by others. Where this is the case, the sense of overall integrity will be high and will enrich the ethical dimension of counselling. This sense of integration may be a goal to work towards, rather than something to be taken for granted. Ultimately, a counsellor's ethical **responsibility** is both personal and professional. But the construction of a personal ethic does not take place in a social vacuum: it is influenced and supported by other ethical sources.

Personal values are important to integrity and resilience as a counsellor but need to be treated cautiously as a basis for resolving ethical dilemmas that relate to clients. Clients' values are more significant than our own for resolving issues that are properly within their **autonomy** or right to self-government. For example, counsellors have to be willing to support clients in making and implementing decisions that they would not wish for themselves or people close to them. A counsellor's personal values are an important platform upon which to build the ethical basis for counselling, but not an adequate basis for ethical decision making on behalf of clients.

Ethics and Values Implicit in Therapeutic Models

Our choice of therapeutic orientation will have ethical implications. Therapeutic models are usually produced to serve therapeutic ends rather than as exercises in secular ethics. Nonetheless, they incorporate ethical orientations and beliefs, usually implicitly. The choice of therapeutic model may be a source of insight into your personal ethical predisposition. A comparison between person-centred and psychodynamic counselling will illustrate this point. Carl Rogers, the founder of person-centred counselling, emphasized the client's capacity for self-determination. Counselling is not viewed as a process of doing something *to* the individual, or inducing them to do something about themselves. Rather, it is freeing the client for personal growth and development and from obstacles so that a move forward can again be achieved. The core conditions of congruence, empathy and unconditional positive regard are simultaneously both an affirmation of client autonomy and a constraint on the counsellor's direct influence on that autonomy. The client is not only assumed to have an innate capacity for growth, but is also the expert on how to achieve this.

In contrast, a Freudian psychodynamic model vests the counsellor with a higher level of expertise in the alleviation of distress in the client, partially through a greater awareness of the influence of the unconscious. The therapeutic theory is based on psychological determinism in which a causal link between past experience and present psychology is assumed. The ultimate goal of achieving client autonomy may be shared with the person-centred counsellor, but the route to achieving that end is different. The counsellor uses an expertise within an ethic of welfare in which responsibility is assumed for assessing what is in the client's best interests in order to alleviate distress and enhance insight. It is also assumed that the trained psychodynamic counsellor is better placed to detect the links between past and present experience than the untrained client.

Other therapies that rely on therapeutic expertise to alleviate distress, such as cognitive, systemic and some humanistic approaches, tend towards an ethic of welfare (i.e. the counsellor knows what is psychotherapeutically best for the client and is required to use that knowledge for the benefit of the client). In contrast, person-centred models and other approaches that are optimistic about the accessibility of personal insights, such as transactional analysis, tend towards an ethic of autonomy (i.e. the client is considered to know what is best for them in the context of their life and experience). Once these associations with different ethical approaches are acknowledged, it becomes much easier to question whether inbuilt ethical biases are appropriate. Person-centred counsellors may find themselves working with clients who, for one reason or another, have considerable difficulty in working within an ethic of autonomy and respond better to a transitional phase in which the counsellor works within an ethic of welfare. Conversely, a psychodynamic counsellor may have a client who is more appropriately counselled within the ethic of autonomy.

The rise of cognitive-behavioural counselling is driven by a combination of values concerning beliefs about the importance of scientific knowledge and evidence in planning publicly funded services and making scarce resources available to the greatest number of people. Brief, time-limited therapy and single-session therapies (Dryden, 2020) may, in part, be more open to other approaches to therapeutic models but typically shares a concern to make the best use of limited resources. However, it is wise not to take the values behind any therapeutic movement as unquestionable truths, and even if those values appear justifiable, they may not match the 'facts' or results of what happens in the implementation of the said values. The facts are often more friendly and mutually inclusive of different therapeutic orientations than any analysis based on differences in values might suggest (Cooper, 2008).

The pluralistic framework, originally proposed by Cooper and McLeod (2010) is based on the principle of self-determination, in that the client is positioned with a frame of autonomy, but also as a collaborative partner in therapy, determining their own integration of therapy that best fits their own needs at that time. Pluralism assumes that no one approach to counselling will be right for every client, all the time. Rather, different people need different things at different times, and the same individual might benefit from one therapeutic approach at one stage, but another at a different time. The place of the counsellor here is to facilitate collaboratively the form and nature of therapy in relation to the tasks and goals agreed at the outset (or developed during the therapy and reviewed).

Overarchingly, values ought not to be taken for granted or adopted unquestioningly. Our preferred choice of therapeutic model and its implicit values provides important insights into ourselves as counsellors, well worth periodic reflection and self-examination. Second, from a client's point of view, the values inherent in our particular approach to therapy will shape their therapeutic journey for good or bad. An unexamined value may become as dangerous or counterproductive as an unacknowledged cause of a client's therapeutic struggle. Unexamined values can set counsellors against their clients just as easily as therapist against therapist. Once value differences can be openly acknowledged and discussed, it becomes easier to find points of human contact and mutual understanding even if agreement cannot be reached. Although the implicit ethical bias of a therapeutic model ought not to be accepted unquestioningly, it is one of the ethical compass points to guide us through the complexities of providing counselling and therapy.

Pause for Reflection

Consider what attracted you to the model you are training in, or have trained in. Was it expediency, in that it was the closest training programme to home, or were there other factors that attracted you to it? What were they and how, as your relationship with your model has progressed, have your model and values informed each other?

Agency Policy

If a counsellor works within an agency, it is commonplace to be required to follow specific protocols and procedures with regard to some ethical and therapeutic dilemmas. For example, many agencies have adopted a policy that child protection takes precedence over individual client **confidentiality**. It is not unusual to find that observance of these policies is a term in the counsellor's **contract** of employment, or that volunteer counsellors are asked to give a written undertaking to observe certain policies.

A precise evaluation of the appropriateness of individual policies will need to take into account the context in which the agency provides its services, its range of clients and their needs, as well as the organizational ethos of the agency. The expansion of the availability of counselling means that it is provided by a whole variety of agencies: some dedicated exclusively to providing counselling, and others where the counsellor may be a single person working alongside several different professions providing a variety of services (e.g. counselling in primary healthcare) or a single profession providing a highly regulated service (i.e. in schools).

Banks (2006) has specialized in ethics for social work and youth workers. She makes a useful distinction between different visions for social work that are increasingly applicable to counselling. Table 3.1 distinguishes between social workers who adopt committed/radical, professional, bureaucratic and quasi-business models of practice; it is possible to see parallel distinctions in counselling. A committed/radical counsellor claims the greatest professional autonomy and **rights** to independent thinking. Most of the pioneers of counselling before the 1980s were of this type. Free-thinking and highly motivated individuals helped to get counselling established as a new movement. However, there was little consistency in how services were delivered or established systems for protecting the **safety** of clients: the best and worst of practice co-existed.

Moves towards introducing professional **standards** were one way of ensuring greater consistency and promoting good practice. Inevitably wherever counselling was delivered within organizations there was the associated bureaucracy of organizational life. Bureaucracy is often viewed negatively as the opposite of creativity, but the right level of skilfully implemented bureaucracy is also essential to the efficient and safe delivery of counselling, particularly as the scale of the service grows. The quasi-business model works by providing competitive services within the marketplace to clients who are viewed as customers. Each of these developments has consequences for counsellor autonomy. The move towards being a profession has placed a greater emphasis on ethical responsibilities to clients in particular. The growth of bureaucracy around counselling is in part a way of evidencing professional **accountability**, but primarily a result of the requirements placed on any organization or business in a developed economy.

At each step, the professional autonomy of the counsellor is reduced in return for providing more credible and **trustworthy** services to the public and in the hope of more consistent opportunities for employment and social recognition of the social value of counselling. To be professional requires **ethical standards**. Being accountable for those standards and working within organizations requires a degree of bureaucracy. However, neither of these developments should be allowed to extinguish the drive and innovative spirit that fired the original visions of counselling as a force for good. To be a force for good each counsellor needs to foster the drive of the radical for improvement, the professional for standards, the bureaucrat for accountability and systems, and the advocate for social justice. As in social work, the tension between these different drives will play out differently in different contexts and organizational cultures.

TABLE 3.1 *Models of practice*

	Committed/radical	**Professional**	**Bureaucratic**	**Quasi-business**
Social work as	vocation/social movement	profession	job	business
Social worker as	equal/ally	professional	technician/ official	producer/ provider
Power from	competence to deal with situation	professional expertise	organizational role	competence in the market
Service user as	equal/ally	client	consumer	customer
Focus on	individual or group empowerment/ societal change	individual worker–user relationship	service provision	customer satisfaction/ profit
Guidance from	personal commitment/ ideology	professional code of ethics	agency rules and procedures	market norms, customer preferences, contracts
Key principles	empathy, genuineness/ raising consciousness, collective action	users' rights to self-determination, acceptance, confidentiality etc.	agency duties to distribute resources fairly and to promote public good	customer choice and independence
Organizational setting that would best facilitate this	independent voluntary agency or campaigning group	private practice or large degree of autonomy in agency	bureaucratic agency in voluntary, statutory or private sector	private agency

Source: Banks (2006) *Ethics* and *Values in Social Work*. Basingstoke: Palgrave Macmillan. (Reproduced with the permission of the British Association of Social Workers and the author.)

Professional Codes, Frameworks and Guidelines

Professional **codes**, frameworks and guidelines are a valuable source of ethical information. They will be the first points of reference for many counsellors. At their best, these documents are a source of collective wisdom validated by a process of consultation during their adoption procedures by the organization that produced them. They often represent a distillation of ethical and legal principles because, even if a code makes no explicit reference to the law, most reputable professional organizations will have sought legal clearance from a lawyer before issuing the code.

However, it is the distilled quality of these ethical statements that is also their greatest limitation.

Codes and ethical **guidance** tend to be written in fairly general and abstract terms in order to condense the experience and thinking behind them and to make them as widely applicable to a variety of circumstances as possible. This means that they are unlikely to be read for their literary quality or narrative pull. Unfortunately, this will discourage some people from reading them in advance of an ethical dilemma and indeed, some members of professional associations that have signed to work within the ethical guidance document of that association sometimes claim never even to have heard of it. This is a pity because the urgency and emotional turmoil surrounding a crisis make this an inauspicious occasion to read a code for the first time. They are complex documents with many interrelated provisions and need to be understood as a whole before the significance of any of the parts can be fully appreciated. Moments of high drama tend to complicate gaining an overall understanding of the contents of a code. Counsellors in an ethical crisis tend to clutch at clauses, as drowning people are said to clutch at straws. Extracted from their context, these clauses of comfort can be quite misleading, especially if that is all that someone is relying on. For example, working with suicidal clients at a point of suicidal crisis often leads counsellors to look for certainty in their ethical frameworks, hoping for a 'tell me what to do' position, and encounter high levels of frustration when they do not find a specific answer. Likewise, however, they can also struggle with a perceived certainty of some policies and procedures which direct them to act in ways counter to their personal values with respect to more general aspects of working with risk (Reeves, 2010).

It is much better to be familiar with relevant codes before a crisis occurs. Often, prior knowledge will enable that crisis to be averted because most ethical guidance forewarns the reader about potential areas of difficulty, and even if the dilemma is not averted this prior knowledge will usually assist in the interpretation of relevant passages.

One rather off-putting characteristic of codes (perhaps the most authoritative form of ethical guidance) is their tendency to be peppered by 'shoulds' and 'oughts'. These directives sit uneasily with counselling and sometimes seem like a professional organization importing a bureaucratic model into a professional ethos that tends to be less authoritarian or collectively minded. The weakening of the authoritative voice in the context of guidance as frameworks is compensated for by greater inclusiveness across human differences and opportunities to take contextual variations into account in resolving ethical challenges.

However, the reality is that any ethical guidance will often be used as the basis for complaints procedures against members of that organization. To breach the terms of a code by which you are contractually bound is a serious matter and can lead to a formal complaint; however, the level of obligation is seldom such to justify blind compliance. That would undermine the ethical basis of the counselling relationship, as it prioritizes the code as being more important than the human relationship. Indeed, there may be occasions when the more ethical response will be to breach the code. Such a breach would only be justified when undertaken in dialogue with supervisors, experienced colleagues and the professional body. To breach a code is a serious matter for which there has to be willingness to be accountable, often within the disciplinary and fitness to practise procedures of the professional body concerned. It is not something to be undertaken lightly without good reason or paying attention to how the decision is reached and implemented.

The ultimate ethical responsibility must rest with the individual counsellor and their personal and professional judgment. Someone who conscientiously breaches a provision of their professional code for carefully considered ethical reasons is in a much better ethical position than someone who breaches a code through ignorance or a reckless disregard for its provisions. Codes, frameworks and guidelines do not eliminate the need for ethical awareness in interpreting how they apply to particular circumstances. It is salutary to remember that most ethical guidance is seldom comprehensive. For example, most counselling codes are relatively silent about working with young people, in comparison to counselling adults, although this area continues to change, with BACP currently developing a competence framework for working with children and young people which sits within a good practice frame (BACP, 2018b, 2019a). Ethical guidance can seldom be definitive. It cannot override legal obligations, at least in the eyes of the law. Guidance is also ephemeral, as all codes are periodically revised and updated in response to changes in social circumstances and working practices. However, there is often a time lag between these developments and their incorporation within the ethical guidance or requirements issued by any professional body.

Moral Philosophy

Moral philosophy is primarily concerned with identifying what constitutes 'good' and 'bad' and using logical reasoning to consider the implications for ethical dilemmas. A subsidiary area of moral philosophy is professional ethics: this is a rapidly growing discipline within moral philosophy, which also draws on other sources from social sciences and the law. The main focus of professional ethics is an interest in the application of core values that constitute an integral part of professional identity.

Medical ethics are probably the most highly developed professional ethics. The long history and academic ethos of medicine have combined to produce some of the most sophisticated approaches to constructing professional ethical systems and in training professionals in how to combine the ethical with technical aspects of their work. Not surprisingly, there is a proliferation of approaches which reflect the diversity of ethical models within moral philosophy. In Europe and North America this has typically taken the form of competition between deontological ethics (i.e. ethics of duty and obligation) founded on the ideas of Immanuel Kant (1724–1804) and utilitarian ethics based on the writing of David Hume (1711–1776), Jeremy Bentham (1748–1832) and John Stuart Mill (1806–1873). The deontological approach is based on deducing ethical obligations from a particular set of beliefs about the nature of reality. These obligations are viewed as universal and can be typified by an emphasis on treating people as ends in themselves. In contrast, the utilitarian approach is founded on an evaluation of the consequences of any action and can be typified by a commitment to achieving 'the greatest good for the greatest number'. The choice between the two systems can be represented as a choice between viewing people as ends in themselves or as means to an end.

The competition between these two ethical approaches has produced several other major responses. One of these has grown out of a critique of the first two as being too founded in the male experience of being an unencumbered individual. This stands in contrast to the female experience of living with the dependency of children, the sick and the elderly. This view of the female experience of ethical responsibility for others has led to the creation of an 'ethic of care', which focuses on the moral implications of the interconnectedness of people. The fourth major approach to current ethics shifts attention from principles to the moral qualities of the person. This has led to a revival of virtue ethics founded on the writing of Aristotle (384–322 BCE), which views ethical action as growing out of personal qualities or virtues and is sometimes also referred to as 'contemplative' ethics. Another approach is not so much a single ethic, but a group of approaches founded on postmodern doubt that it is possible to produce a universal ethic. From this point of view, ethics are, therefore, not defined by the production of a distinctive ethical system but by a commitment to engaging in a mutually respectful discussion from which ethics appropriate to that context can be constructed. These approaches are sometimes referred to as 'communicative' or 'narrative' ethics.

The existence of these different approaches (and many others) has been a major challenge and stimulus to professional ethics in ways that are analogous to the interaction between the major therapeutic traditions within counselling. There have been those who have taken a philosophically strong approach by arguing that one model is both universally applicable and ethically superior to all others. Others have taken a less dogmatic approach and have sought to draw upon aspects of different models appropriate to specific ethical issues and rejected any hastily reached simplicity in ethics. The most influential ethicists of this kind in medical ethics are Tom Beauchamp and James Childress (2019). Their *Principles of Biomedical Ethics*, now in its eighth edition, has had a major influence on the development of ethical principles for counselling and psychotherapy. They propose four major ethical principles:

- **Respect** for individual autonomy (literally self-government).
- **Beneficence** (a commitment to benefiting the client).
- **Non-maleficence** (avoiding harm to the client).
- **Justice** (a fair distribution of services within society).

It is this combination of principles that is most widely referred to in the literature about ethics for counsellors. However, Andrew Thompson, in *A Guide to Ethical Practice in Psychotherapy* (1990), adds a further two principles:

- *Fidelity* (honouring the promises upon which the **trust** between client and counsellor is founded).
- *Self-interest* (the counsellor's entitlement to all the preceding five principles).

The addition of fidelity as a moral principle is highly compatible with counselling and signals the importance of 'trust' and being 'trustworthy'. This seems an obvious addition that increases the relevance of a collection of principles to counselling. In contrast, Thompson acknowledges that the addition of 'self-interest' is controversial. Nonetheless, he argues strongly for the inclusion of this principle by a combination of ethical and psychological reasoning. He takes the view that self-interest is invariably present in ethical decision making and can be a distorting influence when it is left as an unacknowledged factor. The power of unacknowledged factors in personal decision making is much greater when these remain unspoken and therefore have a disproportionate and indeterminate influence on the decision-making process.

The use of a combination of ethical principles as a basis for professional ethics has many strengths. The principles act as vehicles for disseminating a terminology and way of approaching ethical **problems** which take an integrationist approach to many of the major contemporary ethical models. These act as a metaphorical bridgehead between the different disciplines of moral philosophy and counselling. Arguably, they provide counsellors with a greater level of ethical sophistication than they would be likely to develop by simply reflecting on the ethical dilemmas of their role from a purely practical perspective. The usefulness of any model for professionals is determined by a combination of two factors that exist in tension with each other: there needs to be sufficient complexity to accommodate a wide range of applications, but also sufficient simplicity for these to be readily recalled and applied by a busy practitioner. The application of the principles by Thompson has that combination of sufficient complexity and simplicity to be useful to counsellors whose primary concern is not moral philosophy but practical ethics.

The presentation of moral philosophy as principles also matches the bureaucratic needs of professional organizations. Principles provide a convenient method for focusing the membership's attention on the rationale for the collective ethic to which they are bound as well as a readily usable method of **regulation** and adjudication. There is a potentially closer relationship between the expression of individual and collective ethics than would be the case in other approaches to moral philosophy. These positive aspects of the expression of professional ethics in terms of a series of principles have led to some counselling organizations actually promoting them as a method for ethical insight. However, principles are not always easily transferable across cultures.

The New Zealand Association of Counsellors explicitly incorporated these five principles within its *Code of Ethics* (NZAC, 1998) but has downplayed them in later versions (2012, 2020). The explicit adoption of these principles within a code of ethics for counsellors in two very different cultures, white European and Maori, disadvantaged one of them. Principles speak well to a modern westernized **culture** with an emphasis on professional responsibility and reasoning, but can seem to be a strange way of expressing ethics in other cultures. In traditional cultures, virtues or personal moral qualities like loyalty, courage, fairness and wisdom often seem a better way of communicating what matters ethically. Virtues relate to the moral character of someone and also relate to how that person is experienced in their role within a community. Principles relate better to systems and standards that need to be delivered regardless of the particular person undertaking the task, which is why they speak better to professions in modern economies. Interestingly, there has been a revival of interest in virtues in western ethics by revisiting the origins of western ethics in the ideas of Aristotle (384–322 BCE). The revival of virtue ethics may provide a better platform for those of us with European backgrounds to begin to understand and appreciate traditional approaches to ethics. In a global society, we will need a variety of approaches to how we represent and understand ethics in order to appreciate the strengths of each other's cultures and traditions.

Social Justice in Context

The increasing tendency for professional associations and other organizations in the counselling professions to implement the concept of social justice into strategic plans and mission statements is worthy, but also places a challenge to act in accordance with the principles of social justice. Rather than a statement of social worthiness, a true commitment to social justice demands the application of ethical principles in such a way as to challenge and

(Continued)

combat the consequences of social injustice. This, arguably, will inevitably mean that, at times, counsellors – and organizations – act in such a way in order to challenge the status quo and position themselves as advocates for those without power or voice. Is it sufficient to be committed to social justice without a more proactive stance against social injustice?

Law

The **privacy** of most counselling relationships may seem to justify a belief that the law is largely irrelevant to counsellors; this is an illusion. The counsellor and client alike are citizens within a national, and increasingly international, system of law. Being aware of the law has a number of potential gains. Frequently, the law and counselling practice are mutually compatible. A legally well-informed counsellor is best placed to use the law to protect the **rights** and responsibilities associated with their work through a process of supporting self-determination and advocacy. Counsellors seeing fee-paying clients ought to be aware of the law of **contract**, which can be used to support the counselling relationship and clarify both parties' expectations of each other. Ignorance of the law can be correspondingly undermining and introduce unexpected and unwelcome surprises. For instance, in the absence of a clear contractual agreement between client and counsellor, a court may imply a contractual term. Counsellors seeing non-fee-paying clients have greater difficulty in establishing the legal basis of their relationship and may be subject to greater legal uncertainty.

Nonetheless, following the principle that to be forewarned is to be forearmed, all counsellors would be well advised to have at least a basic familiarity with the law concerning contract, **negligence**, defamation, **confidentiality**, the protection and **disclosure** of **records** and acting as a witness (in civil, criminal and coroners' courts) (see Bond and Sandhu, 2005; Mitchels and Bond, 2021). Depending on the type of work undertaken by the counsellor, it may also be appropriate to consider the law concerning mental health, families and young people (see Mitchels and Bond, 2010, 2011). Obtaining this kind of information is becoming progressively easier as new publications appear.

One of the difficulties posed by the law for counsellors is its complexity and the potential for seemingly contradictory legal provisions. Some basic principles of law go a long way towards easing this problem. The law is a hierarchical system. Statute law passed as legislation by Parliament overrides all other kinds of law. In the absence of any statutes, the law may have been created by a system of case law, in which the legal principles developed by the most senior court bind all those below it. Policies adopted by government departments have no legal standing unless they are supported by statute. The courts frequently make the point that government policy by itself is not legally enforceable and that the government has the means at its disposal to make it enforceable, if it be so minded.

It is also important to realize that any contractual term that conflicts with either statute or common law (a form of case law) is unenforceable. This is particularly significant with regard to confidentiality and working with suicidal clients (see Chapters 7 and 10). Another common mistake is to assume that what is good law in one organization automatically applies to all others doing similar work. The legal bases of public sector, commercial and **voluntary** organizations are quite different. Public bodies can only do what they are authorized to do by statute, so may have obligations which would not apply to other kinds of organization. It is also usual to find very different kinds of powers and obligations applying to different public bodies. It is commonplace to find that the legal obligations held by children's services concerning child protection are wrongly thought to apply to other types of organization. As always with the law, the devil is in the detail; the list below attempts to summarize some basic principles for making best use of it.

- Use the most up-to-date law.
- Distinguish between the relevant legislation and case law, as the former overrides the latter.
- Check whether public or agency policy is a legal commitment backed by legislation required by a contract with the people affected.
- Know the terms of your contracts with clients, employers and professional bodies. Ensure that these agree with what you offer your clients.
- Seek advice from a lawyer on important issues.

Pause for Reflection

What ethical issues have you encountered that can arise in counselling? What sources of counselling ethics have been most useful to you in resolving these dilemmas? Why have they been most helpful?

Conclusion

Drawing attention to different sources of ethical insights is useful in counselling to challenge the notion that simply relying on a combination of professional code(s) or guidelines and a sense of personal morality is a sufficient basis for ethical standards in counselling. Codes and guidelines are important, but they are no longer adequate to meet the personal, social and legal challenge that many counsellors may encounter in their work. The law is an increasingly significant source that needs to be taken into account as it represents a form of national morality within a democracy. Moral philosophy provides a basis for re-evaluating many of the 'taken for granted' aspects of the law and professional guidelines, as well as the values implicit within therapeutic models.

When there are so many different sources of ethical insight, how can these be prioritized? Which source carries the authority to overrule the others? The law carries the greatest authority as it is enforceable by courts and is a form of democratically endorsed public morality. The law also takes many forms, including European and national legislation, delegated legislation, and legal principles established from the analysis of cases by the courts. The law applicable to counselling is complex, but is increasingly better understood within the UK. A good starting point is the Legal Resources for Counsellors and Psychotherapists series sponsored by BACP in collaboration with SAGE. The next level of authority is the commitments entered into by counsellors as part of their contractual obligations to clients, employers and professional bodies, as the terms of these contracts need to comply not only with the applicable statutory and case law but also with each other. Contracts that do not comply with state law may be partially or wholly unenforceable and a major source of confusion and misunderstanding.

A much more common source of difficulty arises for counsellors when they have differences between their contractual agreements with their clients and their employers. Typically, these differences will arise when the counsellor promises higher levels of confidentiality to the client than their contract of employment will support. This then often comes to a head when the employer wants information about a client or access to the records, but the counsellor has been working on the basis that confidences are to be kept between counsellor and client. The counsellor is caught between conflicting contractual obligations and a choice of which one to break when breaking either may carry serious consequences. It is so much better to ensure that all contractual commitments, especially to clients and employers, are compatible with each other. For counsellors working in different settings this may mean having to work within different contractual frameworks and obligations. Professional ethics are generally drafted widely enough to encompass a wide range of different contractual commitments, provided clients are properly informed about what to expect from counselling and how their confidences will be managed. State law and contractual obligations set the framework within which ethical judgments have to be made. The most common dilemmas for counsellors concern the protection or disclosure of 'personally sensitive' client information, conflicts of interest, dual relationships and respecting client choices when the counsellor feels strongly that a client could have made a better choice.

As counsellors we are often witness to the moral struggles of our clients as they search for the right thing to do or for moral meaning in what is happening to them. Most of the time the moral dilemma can be appropriately regarded as falling within the client's responsibility, but there will be times when a client's moral dilemma creates the possibility of a professional ethical dilemma for the counsellor. A few examples drawn from suitably disguised real-life events will illustrate this point:

- A school counsellor has been approached by a 13-year-old pupil for counselling about family problems. The pupil's teacher supports the counselling but her parents have expressly forbidden the pupil to receive counselling.
- Connie is seven months pregnant and has deeply held beliefs in favour of natural childbirth and against medical intervention. These feelings are being expressed by a refusal to accept a Caesarean delivery in order to protect both the foetus and herself from the consequences of dangerously high blood pressure. She has no illusions about the seriousness of her situation after nearly dying from similar complications in an earlier pregnancy. She has sought counselling to help her resist increasingly insistent offers of medical help.
- Simon is a student in a residential hall. He had become aware that someone living next door to him is heavily involved in selling illegal drugs because people are knocking on his door in error. He has decided not to report the drug dealing but has requested a transfer of rooms to avoid the disturbance from some quite persistent visitors who call at anti-social hours. The student counsellor who saw Simon is aware that the college is seriously concerned to prevent drug use on its premises but Simon is insisting on confidentiality.

Each of these issues posed complex challenges for the ethical standards of the counsellors concerned which could not simply be resolved by a combination of innate personal morality and the published ethical requirements of their respective professional bodies. A securely based ethical decision needs to take into account insights derived from all the sources considered in this chapter. Counsellors' ability to respond ethically and constructively will be considerably enhanced by the extent to which they have already actively incorporated these sources into the ethical framework that informs their everyday arrangements with clients. The outline of that framework is given in the next chapter.

Pause for Reflection

Consider your response to each of the above scenarios and consider the six sources of ethics discussed, and which aspects you draw on to inform your thinking.

To access the online resources accompanying this chapter, please visit: https://study.sagepub.com/reevesandbond

4

Framework for Counselling Ethics and Standards

Chapter Overview

Much greater consistency has emerged across the variety of professional bodies that operate in the UK. This chapter provides a comparative analysis to identify the major themes that unite the different professional bodies. It concludes with consideration of recent changes in the **regulation** of **counselling** by **statutory regulation** of counselling psychology and accredited **voluntary** registration for counselling and **psychotherapy**.

Key words

ethical framework, **codes**, statutory regulation, **accredited voluntary register**

An ethical framework creates a basic conceptual structure within which we can all feel safe and supported to move around freely and make choices. There is enough of a structure to define the available choices and give a sense of distinguishing what is ethically acceptable from the unacceptable or unwise. This can provide essential support and a sense of direction when feeling overwhelmed with ethical uncertainty. On the other hand, the framework creates sufficient spaces to accommodate legitimate differences of opinion. These are spaces where counsellors can position themselves in ways that fit a sense of personal and professional integrity and take account of clients' needs. The potential for moving around a framework builds in a degree of flexibility that permits changes in position as circumstances change:

> Mutually agreed ethics and acceptable standards of practice in any profession provide the bedrock whereby those practitioners and clients are safeguarded and served within a defined framework and agreed boundaries. In this way the professional search for integrity and credibility is validated. (COSCA, 2014)

This statement draws attention to another aspect of ethical frameworks. These are often the product of collective agreement and endorsed by the members of a profession or professional organization. The most direct sources of the framework are the published **codes** and guidelines. This chapter is primarily based on an analysis of the ethical requirements of five major national **counselling** organizations within the UK and Ireland:

- British Association for Counselling and Psychotherapy (BACP)
- United Kingdom Council for Psychotherapy (UKCP)
- Counselling Psychology Division of the British Psychological Society (BPS)
- Confederation of Scottish Counselling Agencies (COSCA)
- Irish Association for Counselling and Psychotherapy (IACP)

An International Perspective

Codes of **ethics** from the USA, Canada, Australia, New Zealand and Malta have been consulted to identify distinctive **cultural differences** in how ethics are developed for counselling.

Each of these sources of **guidance** has been formally adopted by the professional organization as a set of minimum **ethical standards** that are viewed as important guidance for members. Failing to work within that guidance would be regarded as a legitimate source of concern about the ethical practice of a counsellor, which in serious cases could lead to a disciplinary hearing or their expulsion from membership.

Comparison between the Statements of Ethical Standards

A comparison between the statements of ethics published by the four national associations in the British Isles reveals considerable consensus around the core ethical **issues** for counsellors (see Table 4.1). All the major professional bodies emphasize a number of ethical concerns, and these are:

- client **safety**;
- professional **competence** and fitness to practise;
- **respect** for differences in lifestyles and beliefs between clients;
- respect for client self-determination;
- prohibitions on the **exploitation** of clients;
- contracting;
- confidentiality;
- a duty to maintain the profession's reputation.

TABLE 4.1 *Requirements*

Requirements	BACP	BPS	COSCA	IACP	UKCP
Accuracy in statements about qualifications/professional competence	O	O	I	O	O
Accuracy in advertising and information about services offered	O	O	O	O	O
Therapist competence					
• working within the limits of competence	O	O	O	O	O
• adequate training and experience	O	O	O	O	O
• CPD to update practise	O	O	O	O	O
• regular monitoring and review of practice	O	O	O	O	I
Fitness to practise	O	O	O	O	I
Indemnity insurance					
• membership	O	R		O	O
• accreditation requirements	O				O
Client safety protection	O	O	O	O	O
Respect for client autonomy					
• working with a client's consent	O	O	O	O	O

(Continued)

TABLE 4.1 *(Continued)*

Requirements	BACP	BPS	COSCA	IACP	UKCP
• non-exploitative	O	O	O	O	O
• management of dual relationships	O	O	O	O	O
• non-discriminatory	O	O	O	O	O
Conflicts of interest					
• prohibition of taking on working relationship with clients when there is prior knowledge which might cause a conflict of interest	I	R	O	R	O
Inform client					
• in advance	O		I	I	I
• as soon as apparent	O		O	O	
Take to supervision	O		O	O	O
Equal opportunities and non-discrimination	O		O	O	O
Contracting					
• clarity about terms	O	O	O	O	O
• terms communicated in advance or at outset of working relationship	O	O	O	O	O
• periodic opportunities to review	O		O	O	I
Arrangements for breaks and endings	O		O	O	O
Confidentiality					
Importance emphasized – any limitations to be communicated:	O	O	O	O	O
• in advance	O	O		I	O
• at client's request			I	O	O
Sharing information with other professionals requires:					
• client consent or law requires/permits	O	O	O	O	O
• assessment of client interest	O	O	O	I	O
• endeavour to inform client where appropriate	R	I	O	R	R
• breaching confidentiality only to prevent serious harm to client or others, or when legally required to do so	O	O	O	O	O
Awareness, understanding and consideration of legal requirements and obligations	O	R	O	O	O

Requirements	BACP	BPS	COSCA	IACP	UKCP
Supervision					
• regular	O	W	O	O	O
• ongoing	O	W	O	O	O
• sufficient supervisory arrangements and support					O
Research					
• integrity in treatment of data	O	O		O	
• clarity of agreement with participants	O	O		O	O
• consent required: client has right to refuse participation	O	O		O	O
• participant identity to be protected	O	O		O	
• methods compatible with good standards of counselling and psychotherapy	O	O		R	
Policy about maintaining reputation of profession					
• serious breach of Code of Ethics or Practice to be reported	O		O	O	O
• where colleague's behaviour is detrimental to the profession and the discussion has not resolved matters, report to complaints committee/institute complaints procedure	O	O	O	O	O
Record-keeping	O	O	R	O	O
Work environment					
• avoidance of harassment/discrimination	O	O	I	I	O

Sources: BACP (2018b), COSCA (2014), BPS (2018), UKCP (2019), IACP (2018)

Key: I = Implied; O = Obligatory; R = Recommended; W = Where indicated

Note: As each professional code covers slightly different aspects of therapy, each expressed in different terms, it is impossible to make precise comparisons. This table is simply an interpretative reflection on common themes within these codes of ethics. Some of the organizations produce additional guidance on specific topics (e.g. teaching, supervision, research and other themes) which are not included in this interpretation.

The ethical touchstone around which all other concerns are organized is the client. It is easy to lose sight of the client because much of the content of ethical guidance concerns counsellor behaviour, but this focus on counsellor behaviour is directed to enhancing respect for clients and protecting them from harm. The emphasis on working with a client's consent and prohibitions on the exploitation of clients is a common theme with all the professional bodies. This in turn influences the management of core issues such as contracting with clients and confidentiality, where an emphasis on working with client consent is the established norm on all ethically significant issues unless there is concern about harm to the client or others.

As Table 4.1 has evolved over previous editions of this text, several differences were evident, while now there is very little difference between the professional bodies, which have established robust ethical requirements that set out the ethical standards for their members. Their primary purpose is educational, helping practitioners to know and implement their responsibilities ethically. But they are also documents of last resort that set out the baseline for acceptable practice below which a practitioner may be called to account when someone complains, or in a disciplinary or fitness to practise hearing. It is remarkable that this level of agreement has grown across organizations that sometimes exist in competition with each other and in their origins often sought to be distinctive from one another.

There are probably a number of reasons why this level of consensus between professional bodies in the UK has developed. First, over time all the professional bodies operating in the five nations of England, Scotland, Wales, Northern Ireland and Eire have been governed by European legislation concerning human **rights**, and particularly **privacy** and data protection which are directly relevant to the management of confidentiality as the most frequently raised ethical concern in counselling. In a post-Brexit world of course, the extent to which that legislation will still apply for the four nations of the UK is uncertain; Eire remains in the European Union. There has been a commitment by the UK government to retain the principles of human rights, through the European Convention on Human Rights, signed by the UK in 1950. **Law** carries more authority than ethics however, and thus legislation not only promotes consistency across different countries but also overrules the ethical preferences of different professional bodies.

Professional bodies have also matured over the last 25 years and are therefore more willing to collaborate in the interests of promoting talking therapies. Some members of professional bodies also belong to more than one and therefore draw attention to discrepancies in the requirements between them. Almost all of us will work alongside members of other organizations whom we respect as fellow professionals and view as colleagues with whom we can share ideas about ethics and good practice. Improved transport systems and ease of communication through the internet mean that both counsellors and clients are more aware of how the various professional bodies operate and that may also encourage pressure for greater consistency.

Paradoxically, the expansion of affordable mass-transport systems and ease of communication by **digital** technology and the internet mean that counselling is more exposed to cultural **diversity** around the world. This development raises issues about how counselling accommodates and responds to such diversity, the topic of Chapter 12.

Global Differences to Counselling Ethics

There is more in common between the ethics of the national counselling associations than divides them.

- American Counseling Association (www.counseling.org)
- Australian Counselling Association (theaca.net.au)
- Canadian Counselling and Psychotherapy Association (ccpa-accp.ca)
- New Zealand Association for Counsellors (nzac.org.nz)

Some of the similarities are explained by a shared, if complicated and conflicted, national history of relationships under British rule before claiming independence. This shared history is reflected in a shared language. The ethical challenges and concerns that arise in counselling also appear to be shared. All the themes identified as significant in the comparison between ethical codes in the British Isles feature within these codes, but there is also evidence of distinctive differences in cultural practices:

- *Voice*: There is a clear distinction between rule- and principle-based approaches to writing ethics. This is reflected in length and level of detail. The American Counseling Association has the longest and most detailed of any counselling codes. It is the most rule-based and appears to be written on the assumption that 'what is not forbidden is permitted'. Like all other codes, principles are stated but the application of those principles is spelt out in considerable detail. In comparison all other approaches to ethical guidance are less specific and provide principles to be applied by practitioners. This suggests a cultural difference in expectations of how counsellors are accountable to their professional bodies in complaints and disciplinary procedures. A rule-based system directs attention to the 'letter of the law' and behavioural compliance with what is written, whereas a principled approach is interested in behaviour within the context of the counsellor's reasons for what they did and their motivation. It is the difference between being asked, 'Did you obey?' and 'Can you explain and justify what you did?'
- *Values and principles*: Many of the ethical guidelines state their core ethical commitments as values or principles. There are interesting differences. The Psychotherapy and Counselling Federation of Australia incorporates within their values (Figure 4.1) explicit commitments respecting people's sense of self within their personal and cultural context (PACFA, 2020). The New Zealand Association of Counsellors (NZAC, 2020) is distinctively attentive to the relationship between the first inhabitants, the Maori, and later arrivals, which is reflected in how their values are shaped into principles (Table 4.2).

The fundamental values of Counselling and Psychotherapy are:

- Accountability
- Client focus
- Competence
- Diversity
- Empowerment
- Justice
- Human rights
- Integrity
- Professionalism
- Self-awareness

FIGURE 4.1 *Psychotherapy and Counselling Federation of Australia: Values (PACFA, 2020)*

TABLE 4.2 *New Zealand Association of Counsellors: Values and Principles*

The core values of counselling are:	**Principles: counsellors shall undertake the following:**
3.1 Respect for human dignity	Counsellors shall:
3.2 Partnership	4.1 Act with care and respect for individual and cultural differences and the diversity of human experience.
3.3 Autonomy	4.2 Avoid doing harm in all their professional work.
3.4 Responsible caring	4.3 Actively support the principles embodied in the Treaty of Waitangi.
3.5 Personal integrity	4.4 Respect the confidences with which they are entrusted.
3.6 Social justice	4.5 Promote the safety and well-being of individuals, families, communities, whanau, hapu and iwi.
	4.6 Seek to increase the range of choices and opportunities for clients.
	4.7 Be honest and trustworthy in all their professional relationships.
	4.8 Practice within the scope of their competence.
	4.9 Treat colleagues and other professionals with respect.

Source: NZAC, 2016

New Developments in Counselling Practice

New developments in counselling practice create new ethical challenges. One of the major new developments is the rapid growth of online counselling using a wide variety of means of communication from text messaging to secure chat rooms, webcam, email and the early use of artificial intelligence and online personal 'assistants', for example therapy versions of Siri and Alexa to capture and process assessment information. The internet provides a seemingly endless range of possibilities which opens up counselling to a much bigger variety of providers and users. The ethical challenges involved in the use of new technologies are considered in more detail in Chapter 11.

Conclusion

When a professional body publishes a code or ethical framework, this is usually intended for a wide range of people, agencies and organizations. Any statement of ethics is first and foremost for the benefit of clients whose interests and rights are being drawn to the attention of professionals. Even though the protection of clients' interests is so foundational, it is ironic that they are least likely to read these in advance of receiving counselling. The audience here is made up of the members of the professional body who must commit themselves to observing the ethical guidance as a condition of membership and may be required to be held accountable for any breach in grievance or disciplinary hearings. The third audience is other professionals working alongside counsellors in interdisciplinary teams, who may wish to be informed about the ethical framework to which their colleagues are committed, and the fourth audience is the range of gatekeepers and stakeholders in society, such as politicians, policy-makers and commercial managers, who can determine whether or not particular services ought to be funded as credible and useful contributions to society.

What unites all of these audiences is their concern for the ethical integrity of the service being provided. A published statement of ethical commitment by a professional body on behalf of its membership provides evidence of a collective commitment to being ethical. The degree of consensus across the major professional organizations responsible for counselling in the UK suggests that this commitment is both well established and worked out in a reasonable amount of detail.

However, there are changes in process which will affect the ethical landscape for counselling. One of the difficulties for professional bodies is that they appear to have a conflict of interests between *protecting* the interests of clients and *promoting* the interests of their members, who are the service providers. This becomes very apparent whenever a client has a grievance against a counsellor and wishes to make a complaint or start a disciplinary case. If the professional body is responsible for investigating and deciding the outcome of the grievance, it will be very hard for the client to be convinced that they will get a fair hearing and that the professional body will not 'look after its own'. This is a suspicion that is hard to refute.

The introduction of statutory regulation has changed this for counselling psychologists. It is the regulator, the Health and Care Professions Council (HCPC) in the UK, who will take on primary responsibility for the protection of clients' best interests and those of the professional bodies for the professional development and support of counsellors providing the services. Counselling psychologists are each subject to a statement of duties as a registrant that is set out in the *Standards of Conduct, Performance and Ethics* (HCPC, 2018). The system of regulation for all other counsellors and psychotherapists on accredited voluntary registers by the Professional Standards Authority (PSA) works differently. In this type of regulation, it is the professional body that is accredited to admit people to its own register and to hear complaints and disciplinary cases against registered members. This means that the perception of a potential conflict of interest arising when a profession is hearing complaints against its own members will continue. This system of regulation is still in its early stages of development, so it may be a few years before it is possible to assess the benefits and disadvantages of accredited voluntary registration.

All registrants in both the statutory and voluntary registers are required to maintain their fitness to practise and meet all the other requirements of registration or cease to practise as a counsellor or psychotherapist. Professional bodies will still have a major contribution to make to the support and development of counselling and to the ethical health of the profession beyond the legal requirements of regulation.

Pause for Reflection

What do you look for in ethical guidance from your professional association? Do you consider that the current guidance offers what you need; do you have thoughts about how you might want it to develop further?

To access the online resources accompanying this chapter, please visit: https://study.sagepub.com/reevesandbond

Part II

Responsibility to the Client

5

Safety, Negligence and Insurance

Chapter Overview

What can go wrong that may cause actual harm to clients? This chapter considers some of the obvious and easily overlooked sources of harm. To be forewarned is the best basis for prevention. The chapter concludes with a section on **insurance** as an essential protection for clients.

Key words

physical **safety**, psychological safety, **negligence**, **advice**, insurance

The primary focus of a counsellor's attention is the client, ethically and therapeutically. This means that responsibilities to the client are the counsellor's foremost concern. A key aspect of these responsibilities is to protect the client from any harm that may be caused by attending **counselling**. As we have seen in the previous chapter, the principle of **non-maleficence** (i.e. avoidance of causing harm) is not usually presented as the foremost ethical concern. The published ethical statements of national counselling organizations prioritize more positive ethical principles, which by implication assume that avoidance of harm to the client has been taken into consideration in order to achieve these more positive aims. The aim is not to present a case for prioritizing avoidance of harm over other ethical principles. Reservations about rigidly prioritizing any of the ethical principles over the others would apply equally to this one; however, it is a useful starting point. The potential for causing harm can be avoided or at least substantially reduced by considering in advance how the risk of causing any harm may be obviated or minimized so that the way is cleared for more positive ethical aims.

Client Safety

Counselling is primarily a talking therapy. Therefore, it is relatively easy to overlook the physical dangers and to concentrate on psychological sources of harm. This could be an unfortunate error, affecting not only the client but also the counsellor. It is in the counsellor's own interests to avoid some of the more obvious sources of legal liability, which, if they arose, could result in the payment of substantial damages to a client. Some fictitious examples will provide examples of the kinds of harm that could befall clients.

Physical safety

Bill was so nervous when he entered the **counselling** room that he did not notice a shelf at head level. He bumped his head so badly that he required medical treatment.

The risk of physical injury to a client during counselling is usually fairly low, provided that the counsellor has anticipated any sources of danger and removed them. Nonetheless, there is always the potential for a client tripping, falling off a chair, or bumping into something. In these circumstances the client may seek compensation for any injury, particularly if it appears that the counsellor has not taken sufficient care to protect that client from injury. Normally this claim would be made against the 'occupier', defined in **law** as 'a person who has sufficient control over premises to put him under a **duty of care** towards those who come lawfully upon those premises' (Rogers, 2010). Often this could be the counsellor. Normally the claim would be covered by public liability **insurance** if the counselling is taking place on business or public premises. If the counsellor was held by the court to be in control of the premises and the insurance cover was inadequate, then all or part of the claim might have to be met by the counsellor personally. This has important implications for both counsellor and client. If Bill's injuries were serious or resulted in **disability**, any award for damages could be substantial. Figure 5.1 demonstrates a counselling session where several hazards and unprofessional behaviours are evident.

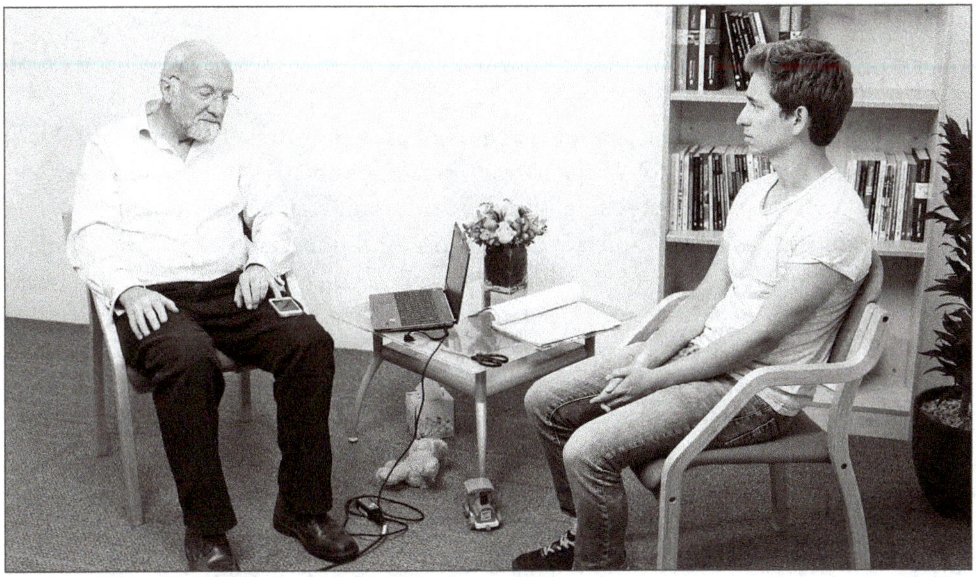

FIGURE 5.1 *Spot the errors**

Many counsellors work from home and may be relying on their household insurance for protection. The counsellor's household insurance company should always be fully informed because failing to inform the insurer about working from home could potentially invalidate an existing household policy. Also, most household insurance policies exclude cover of premises, or parts of premises, used for business purposes, and when informed that a counsellor is working from home, they may refuse cover, impose conditions or charge an additional premium.

Without adequate insurance cover for public liability, a counsellor could be personally liable to pay damages. It is therefore important, whatever the circumstances of working, that a counsellor seeks **advice** from a competent insurance broker about whether 'public liability insurance' is a requirement.

*Mobile phone; trip hazards; scissors; confidential client papers

Pause for Reflection

Have you considered the physical space in which you work and the potential hazards that might exist for your client's physical safety?

Online safety

While online counselling (e.g. via email, chat or video platforms) has been established for some time, the COVID-19 pandemic in 2020 saw many counsellors having to suspend face-to-face counselling and move into an online environment. While organizations such as BACP and the Association for Counselling & Therapy Online (ACTO) have provided excellent guidance for many years, counsellors often focused on the transition of the therapeutic relationship to an online environment and less attention was given to the space of the online world. In a face-to-face setting, counsellors often spend a great deal of time ensuring the physical space is conducive to therapy, but perhaps less so for the online space. The potential for self-disclosure (family photos, other aspects of a counsellor's private world) is greater when online sessions are delivered from a living room, or bedroom (where they would not ordinarily be), or where there may be intrusion of other family members. While much humour surrounded television interviewees being interrupted by their children, such an event in a counselling session could be profoundly distressing for a client.

Likewise, the counsellor needs to ensure that they inform themselves of online safety, including the security of the technology platforms they use, and that sufficient attention is given to encryption, for example. In the early days of the pandemic many trainers, new to an online setting, struggled to successfully implement appropriate security settings to safeguard the integrity of the training session, or found that security offered by platforms at that time were insufficient for their needs. The online space of counselling requires commensurate care and attention, in the same way as a physical space for face-to-face therapy would be. Ethical frameworks (ACTO, 2020) and good practice (BACP, 2019b) are an excellent starting point for this and, of course, additional training.

Psychological safety

All the counselling models of theory and practice claim that clients will benefit from counselling and usually favour a particular theory and method. Working with clients is seldom as straightforward as the counselling models suggest. There will be moments when a counsellor will be faced with making difficult choices about how to respond and assessing what will be most helpful for a client. Especially in the early stages of a counselling relationship, it is often possible to sense a client's vulnerability around issues that have not yet been declared. It then takes time for the necessary **trust** to develop which will enable the client to voice that vulnerability. There can often be differences between trainees and experienced counsellors in their confidence in allowing a client space to move into vulnerable areas. Inexperienced counsellors are more likely to feel the burden of having to be seen to have something to offer and therefore become more challenging in their interventions than a client's level of trust can sustain.

Fortunately, most clients are sufficiently resourceful to protect themselves against such psychologically mistimed interventions whether from inexperienced or experienced counsellors. However, it is unethical to rely on this capacity for self-protection. Any process with the potential for good is likely to have the potential for harm when it is misapplied. In medicine, a subsidiary principle to non-maleficence has been adopted for situations when it is considered that no further help is possible or it is unclear how helpful a particular intervention will prove to be: 'Above all, do no harm.' This sense of **respect** for a client's situation and proper caution in assessing the appropriate way of responding to the client is fundamental to psychological **safety** and thus serves both ethical and therapeutic aims. All the published requirements of professional organizations considered in the previous chapters stress that counsellors should work within their level of **competence**, which is clearly an essential requirement for avoiding client harm. The use of counselling **supervision** where these issues can be discussed remains an additional safeguard for clients.

The ethical significance of avoiding psychological harm to a client is barely matched by the corresponding legal obligation. The example below will illustrate the sort of situation in which a claim for compensation for psychological harm could arise and the difficulties clients may encounter in obtaining damages.

Peter approached a counsellor for assistance with a bereavement. Despite the counselling, he felt progressively worse and became more withdrawn. Eventually he was treated for depression by a psychiatrist. On his recovery, he considered suing his counsellor.

If a counsellor has created a **contract** with a client promising improvements or the absence of deterioration, that client could sue for breach of contract. However, Cohen (1992) observed that:

> counsellors and psychotherapists wisely, therefore, tend to be very cautious about predicting outcomes, and the very wisest of them promise nothing at all! Some who do choose to make extravagant claims for their brand of counselling or therapy offer no quibble money back guarantees to disappointed clients: this is a sensible precaution against claims for misrepresentation and breach of contract.

This advice from one of the first lawyers to take an interest in legal issues for counsellors remains highly relevant to current practice.

In the absence of any contractual terms relevant to a claim, a client's case would be based on the alleged **negligence** of the professional concerned, in this case a counsellor. In order to establish their case, a client would need to show the existence of:

- a duty of care;
- a breach of that duty;
- proof that damage was caused by this breach of the counsellor's duty of care (the causal link).

The level of the **duty of care** owed by counsellors is the same as that of any other professional. They are required only to exercise reasonable care and skill in rendering their services to clients. The duty of care does not require that there should be no deterioration, or even that there should be actual improvement. Reasonable care will be assessed by a court via an examination of the **standards** of the profession, particularly its guidelines about **ethics** and conduct, its leading textbooks and the testimony of its leading practitioners. If, as is the case in counselling, there are differences in view about what constitutes acceptable professional behaviour (e.g. variations between theories and methods of counselling), these will pose a problem for the court. In such circumstances, the court does not become involved in assessing which treatment is more effective, and nor does it regard less effective treatments as negligent. (This could be significant in view of the current **evidence-based practice** guidelines discussed in Chapter 16.)

An assessment of effectiveness would be fraught with **problems** and would leave no room for differences of opinion between conscientious and generally competent practitioners. Courts have therefore adopted a different approach, which is that professional practice is not considered to be negligent if it follows the practice accepted at the time as proper by a reasonable body of professional opinion skilled in the particular form of treatment (Rogers, 2010). The test used to decide whether this is the case was formulated in *Bolam v Friern Hospital Management Committee* (1957), which covered medical negligence, but now has much wider application. Kenneth Cohen (1992) has indicated the kind of question that a judge might ask themself:

> Even though there is a body of competent professional opinion which might adopt a different technique, did the practitioner act in accordance with a practice accepted as proper by a responsible body of professional opinion skilled in the particular form of treatment?

If counsellors can show that they acted in accordance with a reasonable body of competent professional opinion, then there is likely to be a complete defence, but there are still uncertainties about how counsellors would establish this defence. Courts already attach great weight to medical opinions, but the status of non-medical opinions is increasing, where that opinion is given by someone who is sufficiently qualified and experienced to be viewed as an expert witness. Increasingly, courts will also refer to official guidelines for practice, such as those from the National Institute for Health and Care Excellence (NICE), Improving Access to Psychological Therapies (IAPT, 2020), ethical **guidance** from a relevant professional body (e.g. the BACP's *Ethical Framework*, 2013/updated), and authoritative sources about the professionally endorsed variety of approaches to providing counselling.

In order to succeed, a client must also establish that the breach of the duty was the cause of the harm suffered. 'Cause' is defined strictly to mean 'materially contributing' rather than 'determining'. This means that conjectural and speculative explanations of the cause of the harm are inadequate. The question may be put as 'Would the loss or harm have happened but for breach of this duty?' The existence of more than one possible explanation, particularly explanations not involving the counsellor, could discredit or reduce the claim. In Cohen's opinion, there may also be an inherent anti-litigation bias within counselling arising from the difficulty a client has in establishing a counsellor's **responsibility** for the harm suffered in a relationship where the client retains a high level of responsibility for the outcomes of the counselling: 'Many would say that in the long run, a good counsellor or therapist seeks to empower and encourage his client to locate causality operating in her life more and more within herself, rather than others, including in particular the counsellor' (Cohen,1992). Although the law has continued to develop since he made this observation, this is still generally true. On the other hand, an empowered client might become more active in pursuing grievances against the counsellor if that individual has been negligent in the way they have worked.

There are other legal rules that may adversely affect a client's ability to sue for negligence. No compensation is available for hurt feelings alone in this kind of case unless they are of sufficient duration and severity to amount to mental **illness** (see *McLoughlin v O'Brian* [1983] 1 AC 410 at 431) and recent cases have affirmed this general principle.

A client is likely to experience considerable difficulties in bringing a legal action against a counsellor for negligence resulting in psychological harm. This raises the question about whether professional organizations and any agencies providing counselling have a responsibility to hear complaints that receiving counselling has caused serious personal harm. Most of these bodies will hear allegations of harm arising from clearly unethical behaviour, such as the sexual or financial **exploitation** of clients, but are less likely to consider issues relating to poor practice. It is noticeable that the medical profession is moving fairly rapidly towards creating systems that compare the outcomes of different practitioners by systems of clinical audits and are increasingly concerned to respond to complaints about poor practice. There are significant difficulties in providing these kinds of service even within the relatively regulated world of medicine, and these difficulties are likely to be greater within counselling. Nonetheless, there is a strong ethical case for establishing parallel procedures for counsellors, which is strengthened by the near impossibility of bringing successful legal claims for negligence. All PSA accredited register holders, such as BACP, UKCP and the National Counselling Society (NCS) for example, have developed disciplinary and complaints procedures. All registrants on either statutory or **accredited voluntary registers** are potentially subject to disciplinary or fitness to practise procedures.

In the case of *Landau v Werner* (1961) it was held that the defendant, a psychoanalytically orientated psychiatrist, was liable for negligently causing deterioration in his client's condition by engaging in social contacts with her in a misguided attempt to resolve her transference. Her deterioration had been such that she attempted **suicide**. The Court of Appeal upheld this High Court judgment. Both courts rejected allegations that the defendant had had sex with his client.

The lack of cases against counsellors based on negligence is in sharp contrast to the USA, where the rules for establishing liability are much more favourable to the client and therefore litigation is a much more frequent occurrence. For a more detailed exploration of the law of negligence see Mitchels and Bond (2010) *Essential Law for Counsellors and Psychotherapists*, and Jenkins (2007) *Counselling, Psychotherapy and the Law*.

Inappropriate Advice

One of the ways in which clients can be harmed is by being given inappropriate or misleading advice. There are a variety of approaches to the appropriateness of giving advice within counselling. Historically, members of the BACP have striven to distinguish counselling from advice-giving. For over a decade the BAC (the forerunner of the BACP) provided ethical guidance that 'Counsellors do not normally give advice' (BAC, 1997: B.1.3.6). This is probably generally true of all counsellors when it is applied to matters like a decision about leaving a partner, which is usually a personal matter that falls within client autonomy (see Chapter 6). However, models vary in the extent to which they consider it appropriate for counsellors to give advice or be directive about the counselling. There is some research evidence that counsellors use other types of communication strategy to influence clients, even when they claim to avoid advice-giving (Silverman, 1996). There is also an ethical case for creating an obligation on counsellors to advise clients about the potential risks of seeking counselling where these are reasonably foreseeable by a counsellor.

Some models of counselling have no reservations about the value of giving advice and advocate constructive directions to clients that might include undertaking specified exercises or activities such as 'homework' between sessions. Cognitive behavioural therapy and many forms of brief therapy take a positive view of appropriate advice-giving. One of the keenest advocates of advice within therapy and counselling was the late Albert Ellis (1913–2007), who asserted the value of talking clients into something that he believed on theoretical and practical grounds would be therapeutic. He was critical of counsellors who avoided challenging inappropriate or self-destructive beliefs, and argued that the timidity of a counsellor colluded with the client's own maleficence towards themselves (Dryden, 1998). Ellis was an energetic advocate for rational emotive behavioural therapy (REBT), the model of which he was the founder and which has influenced other approaches to cognitive therapy. His views directly opposed the established practice of person-centred and psychodynamic approaches to counselling where abstinence from advice-giving has been much more the norm. It could be argued, however, that professional ethics need to avoid being partisan about ways of working that are considered to be valuable within established therapeutic approaches. It would be as wrong to require that counsellors give advice as to require that they abstain from giving advice. The ethical case for giving advice which is consistent with a chosen counselling model is a strong one. In the context of a model which depends upon advice-giving, a counsellor's deliberate avoidance of doing so may harm a client by withholding a potential benefit of counselling and violate the basis on which that client is seeking counselling. In addition, there is another situation where there is probably a general duty on all counsellors to consider giving relevant advice. This concerns informing clients about any potential risks of counselling.

John is a student who is shortly to sit important examinations. He is actively anxious about taking the exams and this anxiety is compounded by a sense that the current stress has re-stimulated early childhood traumas.

It is not unusual for people who are facing major life events also to experience a resurgence of feelings from other aspects of their life, which seem to compound their difficulties. The challenge for counsellors is finding ways of responding constructively to those life events, such as the forthcoming examination in the example, and assessing whether dealing with the other aspects of clients' issues would be better undertaken before or after their current challenging life event. It is increasingly usual practice among student counsellors to be cautious about starting major counselling work close to examinations. There is a strong ethical case for advising a client to consider dealing with those issues after the examination has been completed, and to keep the focus of the counselling on managing the immediate anxiety about the examinations. At least the client ought to be alerted to the possibility that the emotional demands of dealing with other issues simultaneously with a major life event may reduce their level of energy and ability to focus on that life event.

It may also be ethically appropriate to advise someone to seek specialist help other than counselling or in parallel with counselling. For example, someone may present with constant headaches and a loss of co-ordination, which they then attribute to stress-related problems. Such symptoms could equally well indicate a physical illness such as a brain tumour, where early diagnosis can be critical to the outcome of any treatment. It is ethically appropriate to advise such a client to seek a medical examination to eliminate the physical origins of symptoms or to clarify the nature of the counselling task. Most counsellors' lack of medical training increases the ethical case for maintaining clear **boundaries** as regards the responsibility for physical and psychosocial issues. People with eating disorders are often reluctant to seek medical help and yet severe forms of eating disorders can have long-term consequences for health and fertility and can be life-threatening. Again, this is a situation where a counsellor may wish to advise medical checks in parallel with the counselling. It would be inappropriate for a non-medically trained counsellor to be monitoring weight loss, but where this is an issue there are good ethical reasons for at least advising about the consequences of not seeking that kind of help.

The law recognizes the potential harm caused by negligent advice (sometimes referred to as 'negligent misstatement') and makes the tests for legal liability less stringent than for negligence. Unlike in the action for negligence where a client would have to prove a direct causal connection between the breach of a duty of care and the harm (see the previous section), in negligent misstatement a client would simply need to show that a counsellor took professional responsibility for the advice given, and that the client acted in reliance on that advice to their detriment. Unlike claims for personal injury in negligence, the client would also be able to claim for purely economic losses (e.g. a loss of earnings suffered as a result of bad advice), even though there might have been no damage to person or property and/or no legally recognized contractual relationship between counsellor and client. However, there is no liability for advice given informally, for example in a discussion at a social event for which a counsellor took no professional responsibility (Rogers, 2010).

Negligence in the context of counselling practice might take several forms: for example, a serious lack of empathy, overstepping boundaries in the relationship with a client, failing to recognize serious mental illness or suicidality, or giving inadequate or incorrect advice in the context of a modality where advice-giving is the norm. A counsellor's failure to meet their duty of care and their consequent potential liability for negligence in tort will be the same in all these cases.

Counsellors who advise homework for clients (as opposed to facilitating clients setting their own homework between counselling sessions) may incur liability if there is a breach of a duty of care and clients act on the advice to their detriment. Cohen (1992) gives two speculative examples:

> Suppose … a client says in effect: 'I confronted my boss as we agreed I would. But now he's fired me and I wouldn't have lost my job but for your bad advice.' Or suppose a client is arrested by the police for engaging in sexual activities which his counsellor had negotiated with him as homework without realising they are illegal.

These examples illustrate the legal risks of advice-giving and how poor or wrong advice can be deemed negligent in law.

There is a general principle in medical negligence law that failing to advise the risks of treatment can be as negligent as giving bad advice (*Sidaway v Bethlem Royal Hospital*, 1985). However, counsellors are in a different position from that of medical advisers. They are not usually providing medicines with known potential side-effects or performing physical procedures which often involve some degree of risk, which are recognized by a body of professional opinion that considers such risks ought to be disclosed. The risks of counselling will depend upon each client's specific circumstances, and the nature and degree of risk may vary as counselling progresses (e.g. if a client has unexpected big life events to face, or suddenly becomes psychotic or suicidal). Some clients may need warnings at some point in their therapeutic process; others may never require one. There is no general duty to provide warnings, but in any counselling alliance a situation may develop in which a therapist has a duty to warn a client, and that duty will depend upon the client's particular circumstances.

The Importance of Insurance

It is a requirement for all registered counsellors (regardless of the type of register or professional body) to have adequate indemnity **insurance** in their personal capacity or through their employer. The risk of legal action against a counsellor is relatively small, which is usually reflected in proportionately small premiums. However, the costs have been considerable where counsellors have been held liable for matters such as clients falling and injuring themselves (public liability), malpractice, errors and omissions (professional liability), or other sources of harm to clients. Professional indemnity insurance (to cover professional liability) and public liability insurance are both necessary. Damages in major physical injury cases, usually arising from car accidents, can exceed £5 million, and exceptionally can reach £10 million for a lifetime of 24-hour intensive care. Such severe levels of injury are unlikely to happen as a direct consequence of counselling.

However, no counsellor can be totally confident that a client will not slip on stairs or trip up on a carpet or rug and receive chronic injuries. Whether the injury arises directly as a result of the counselling or is the counsellor's responsibility as the occupier of the premises, it is ethically desirable that the client can be as adequately compensated as possible. The legal purpose of damages awarded to clients in these circumstances is to put them in as good an economic position as if the accident had not occurred. The person who is adjudged to be liable is often responsible for paying both parties' legal costs. Whatever the shortcomings of a rather slow and cumbersome legal process, these are ethically desirable aims. The most practical way of achieving these ethical objectives is through insurance or membership of a professional protection society, unless the counsellor has enormous personal resources to indemnify themself. It is recommended that an adequate policy should include:

- professional liability indemnity (malpractice, errors and omissions);
- public liability cover (including occupier's liability);
- libel and slander insurance;
- product liability cover (particularly relevant to counsellors who supply items such as relaxation tapes and CDs);
- cover for complaints made against the counsellor to professional bodies and regulators.

There is now a good choice of providers who advertise in professional journals or can be identified by internet searches.

For further information about indemnity and other types of insurance, see Chapter 6 in Mitchels and Bond (2010) *Essential Law for Counsellors and Psychotherapists.*

The case for having adequate insurance is not simply altruistic, on behalf of the clients. There is also a degree of self-interest. Even the costs of preparing a legal defence to a relatively minor claim can run to several thousands of pounds, which may be prohibitively expensive for an individual counsellor. The payment of relatively modest premiums provides a degree of financial safety for the counsellor as well as protection for the client.

To access the online resources accompanying this chapter, please visit: https://study.sagepub.com/reevesandbond

6

Respect for Client Autonomy

Chapter Overview

Respect for client **autonomy** – the right to be self-governing in whatever way that is understood by a client – is at the heart of **counselling ethics**. This chapter explores different approaches to respecting client autonomy adopted by well-respected counsellors before considering the ethical challenges encountered in everyday practice. These include: the client forced to receive counselling; providing sufficient information to inform the client's choices; the importance of contracting; and differences in **values** and beliefs between counsellor and client.

Key words

autonomy, self-government, **voluntary**, contracting, personal values, faith, racist, sexist

Respect for client **autonomy** is a high priority in most approaches to **counselling**. Without a commitment to respect for client autonomy or self-determination, counselling would become an ethically compromised and potentially self-diminishing activity for clients. Counselling involves a client being invited to engage in a particular kind of self-talk by a counsellor trained in how to draw someone into this sort of personal reflection. A client is wise to be cautious about engaging in this kind of activity as it will have potentially major implications for that person's sense of **identity** and choice of actions. Counselling is also taking place in circumstances where power is unevenly distributed between counsellor and client, in favour of the counsellor. Especially in the early stages of a counselling relationship there is an inherent inequality between the person seeking help and the person offering help. It is arguable that current trends towards professionalization increase that inequality by adding the weight of collective authority to that held by the counsellor as a person. In the absence of a strong and firmly rooted ethic of respect for individual autonomy, the client could be subjecting themself to manipulation according to the counsellor's agenda or for other purposes. As most people seek counselling at a time of personal difficulty, they are more than usually vulnerable, and therefore counsellors' professional ethic needs to be correspondingly conscientious about respecting client autonomy.

Autonomy means the right to 'self-rule' or 'self-government'. Gillon (1985) has provided a more personally meaningful definition which identifies the essential characteristic as 'the' capacity to think, decide and act on the basis of such thought and decisions, freely and independently and without, as it says in the passport, 'let or hindrance'. However, an emphasis on client autonomy poses several major challenges for the counsellor: how does the counsellor manage the seemingly contradictory expectations of respecting client autonomy while being a constructive influence for the client?

One of the means of resolving the dilemma is to work in ways that enhance client autonomy. This seemingly simple strategy conceals the difficulty of what this might entail, which is probably best illustrated by the various metaphorical labels used by counsellors and therapists to describe how they work. This is an issue on which counsellors, recognized for their personal and professional integrity, hold quite different views without necessarily rejecting the importance of client autonomy.

In a seminal book about *Therapists' Dilemmas*, Dryden (1998) interviewed 14 well-known therapists and counsellors about the challenges of their work and especially those issues which were hard to resolve. A recurrent theme was the challenge of representing accurately the boundary for counsellor and client responsibilities. Many of the interviewees used imagery and metaphors in order to help them describe their dilemmas. It might be helpful to reflect on the differences of view expressed by Albert Ellis, the founder of rational emotive behavioural therapy (REBT), and John Bancroft, a psychiatrist and the author of *Human Sexuality and its Problems* (1989). Ellis conceived the role of therapist as 'scientific healer' with characteristic personal vigour. When interviewed by

Dryden he commented on the situation where a practitioner knows the solution to a client's problem:

> [W]hy should you waste therapeutic time collaborating 50–50 with the clients when you can effectively help them zero in on what their philosophic problems are? ... Indeed, if you do try to maintain a fully collaborative stance, I think you are adopting a hypocritical pretence ... My hypothesis is that many therapists, who are scared shitless of making mistakes in therapy, like 'full collaboration' because they can cop out of taking risks and of doing a great deal of the therapeutic work themselves ... They are, in a word, afraid of being directive. (Quoted in Dryden, 1998: 13)

Ellis believed that it was desirable that therapists would try to fit clients into their system, as opposed to modifying their system to fit clients. He also asserted that it was legitimate to try to talk clients into something that he believed on theoretical and practical grounds was therapeutic. The degree of autonomy he granted clients was the right to consent to therapy on these terms, or to refuse to be persuaded and choose someone else as their therapist. He was advocating a view of the counsellor as holding authoritative expertise based on evidence and professional reflection.

In contrast, Bancroft experiences the dilemma of being both a 'healer' and an 'educator' quite acutely. He acknowledges the attractions of being a 'healer' and that this image can be effective, particularly in the short term, but he cannot escape from being the 'expert' and implying the message 'This is what you should do'. He argues that the disadvantage of the healer role arises at the end of the therapy. He comments about his work with couples as follows:

> If they leave a course of counselling thinking that they have been 'treated', then they are not going to see themselves as equipped with new resources to deal with problems that may arise in the future. So, it is a very important part of my 'educator' role to get the couple, by the time they have left me, to have a clear understanding of what has happened, why it has been helpful, so they can apply these principles themselves. (Quoted in Dryden, 1998: 19)

He has observed that the association of 'healing' with 'expert' and 'higher dependence' also contributes to a higher rate of relapse following counselling. In contrast, an educator who acts in the role of 'guide' fosters a greater sense of self-reliance with a lower rate of relapse.

Pause for Reflection

Given the views of Ellis and Bancroft, what are the implications for the extent of counsellor responsibility from each perspective, and how might that inform your own sense of yourself as a counsellor in relation to your client's autonomy?

Respecting client autonomy within the counselling process cannot be resolved simply by following a set of rules or guidelines, such as abstaining from advice-giving. There may be other good reasons for abstaining from advice-giving, especially where it is inconsistent with the therapeutic approach being used, but this does not make all advice-giving inappropriate. Respecting client autonomy makes greater demands on counsellors. It requires communication with a level of authority and personal challenge appropriate to a particular client at that point in the counselling relationship. One factor which a counsellor might wish to take into consideration is the balance between the level of trust that exists between them and the level of challenge that the counsellor offers.

Social Justice in Context

A level of challenge appropriate to a well-established and secure counselling relationship might be profoundly disrespectful, if not bullying, with another client where the relationship is less secure and the level of trust is insufficient to enable the client to counter-challenge the counsellor or express reservations. A counsellor's role is to enhance a client's capacity for personal autonomy, on whatever level that exists. But this will also be shaped by many factors that sit outside of the counselling room, including poverty, discrimination and other aspects that might undermine the client's sense of self.

Subjectively, people experience their own sense of autonomy quite differently, according to the general circumstances of their life and the dynamics within specific relationships. A loss of confidence, feeling deskilled or being unable to say what one really wants to communicate can all be assisted by counsellors actively working towards enhancing client autonomy. The essential requirement is respecting each client's own sense of what will be helpful to them, whether this involves presenting a choice and accepting that a client may prefer to seek help elsewhere rather than follow the counsellor's recommendations or carefully constructing a mutually agreed basis for working together.

A particularly potent combination, which can undermine client autonomy, can arise when counsellors believe that they know what is best for clients better than clients do for themselves, and this is reinforced by counsellors' determination that clients should comply with their prescription. This determination most commonly arises when a counsellor gains satisfaction from exercising power and control over others or zealously wants a client to conform to their own personal experience or a particular theory.

Sue's partner has recently died. Her counsellor frustrates her by appearing to expect that the same things that helped the counsellor in a similar situation will also help Sue. Sue also finds that the way she is expected to follow a series of stages in her grieving, which do not fit her experience, is unhelpful. This situation could resolve itself in several ways: Sue could lose confidence in her own experience and start to conform to her counsellor's personal and theoretical expectations (this is clearly a move away from autonomy towards dependency); she could abandon the counselling as unhelpful (an opportunity would be lost); or she could challenge the way in which the counsellor is working (a risky thing to do and she may not have the emotional energy for this course of action when she is feeling so vulnerable). The best outcome is that the counsellor is sensitive to Sue's reactions and invites her feedback, and perhaps with the help of counselling supervision modifies her approach, thus demonstrating respect for Sue's personal experience and her autonomy.

This example demonstrates the power held by counsellors over vulnerable clients and how, through too great an enthusiasm for a particular theory or approach, autonomy can be eroded and a client's dependency inadvertently be encouraged. The example given assumes that the client has sufficiently developed insight to be able to recognize what is happening and has the capacity to take the initiative. Other clients may be so used to having their experiences invalidated that they will fail to recognize what is happening to them. The counsellor is then in a very powerful position and this is dangerous unless they are aware of the possibility of using that power to undermine the development of client autonomy. Miller (1998) characterizes such situations as potentially 'poisonous'. She is especially concerned with the way orthodox psychoanalysis dismissed clients' accounts of childhood sexual abuse as fantasy.

Psychoanalytic theories had the effect of automatically, and unconsciously, acting as blinkers which excluded from view the real experiences of a client's childhood. Almost all counsellors would now accept the possibility that the client may be recalling actual events when they describe childhood sexual abuse. The widespread acceptance of this point of view took place in the 1980s. However, it is salutary to wonder whether there are other theoretical 'truths' in a counsellor's repertoire which blinker them against the client's experience. It is important not to exclude something from view that needs to be taken as true if a client's right to act autonomously is to be respected rather than poisoned by a counsellor's disbelief or interpretation. This is not an ethical argument against theory or making interpretations. It is an argument for avoiding investing theories with too much certainty and attempting to impose a point of view on a client, especially if it contradicts the client's reported experience. Both clients and counsellors need a degree of emotional health in order to recognize these situations. In Miller's words, 'Only a feeling person can grasp the way an empty theory may function as a means of power, for he or she will not be intimidated by incomprehensibility' (1998: 8).

Respecting Boundaries in Counselling

The interviews in Dryden's *Therapists' Dilemmas* (1998) suggest that counsellors are most forcefully confronted with what is the appropriate boundary of responsibility in either of two situations. The first arises when a counsellor believes that they can see a solution to a client's problems that has not yet occurred to that client, for example by thinking 'This problem could be solved by doing ...'. The second occurs when a client asks a counsellor to express a personal opinion such as 'Do you think my relationship is dead?' or 'Do you think I am capable of overcoming this problem?' These situations arise frequently in counselling and are often best solved by counsellors asking themselves:

- Am I as counsellor taking on responsibilities that are more properly the client's?
- Is there a way I could respond that maximizes the client's autonomy and minimizes their dependence on me?

These answers help to identify 'where the boundaries lie between counsellors' and clients' responsibilities'. Counsellors who systematically ask themselves these questions are much more likely to stay within boundaries that give clients appropriate responsibility for the outcome of the counselling.

Pause for Reflection

What active steps do you take in your counselling to consider boundaries and autonomy and where responsibility sits in the process for change?

Good practice that respects client autonomy will always involve building clients' capability to make choices and take actions that they consider right for themselves. Poor practice would involve overriding the boundary between a counsellor's and client's responsibilities to interfere in what are properly the client's responsibilities. Even when the intention is positive and the client might benefit from the intervention, the overall effect of crossing boundaries is to erode a client's capability and increase their dependency on the counsellor. This runs against the aims of counselling, which are always to promote clients' control of their own lives in ways that are meaningful to them.

Boundary violation

Fred is talking about the stress caused by not knowing what is going to happen to his work and his fear about whether he is about to lose his job. What would be bad practice? What would be good practice?

Respect for clients' boundaries honours many of the principles of being trustworthy and recognizing client autonomy. Building clients' capacity to control and act in their sphere of influence is a fundamental characteristic of counselling that sets it apart from other types of helping relationships, including friendship and being a parent. Friends and parents may assume the authority to know someone's wishes or what is best for them in ways that counsellors would deliberately avoid in order to build their clients' sense of being in control on the basis of understanding themselves better. Developing insight and building the confidence to act for oneself are core aims in all approaches to counselling. Counsellors' attention to boundaries involves the following:

- *Distinguishing between the process and outcome of counselling*: The counsellor takes responsibility for managing the counselling process but clients are responsible for the outcomes of the counselling in their lives. This means that counsellors avoid claims like 'I cured …' or 'I improved my client's relationships with …'. These are things that the client achieves. Effective counselling creates the conditions that make these outcomes possible for the client to achieve.

- *Maintaining the* ***privacy*** *and* ***confidentiality*** *of counselling*: This is in order to put a client in the greatest possible control of their life without the counsellor providing information that changes the circumstances or interferes with things that are properly the client's responsibilities.
- *Avoiding conflicts of interest*: This maintains a firm focus on the client's autonomy and best interests.
- *Managing dual relationships carefully by paying attention to the implications for counselling*: Dual or multiple relationships involve counsellors being in more than one role in relationship to clients. It is widely considered better to avoid dual relationships whenever this is possible as the easiest way of protecting boundaries from actually (or even the suspicion that they may be) being crossed inappropriately. However, it is recognized that this is not always possible or even desirable in some circumstances. A counsellor who lives with integrity and shows respect in their routine interactions in their community will be much more likely to be trusted to treat clients with integrity and respect. A dual relationship in which a counsellor holds a position of authority over a client (e.g. as an assessor, manager or employer) would be very difficult to manage in ways that would maintain boundaries that respected client autonomy, and this would usually be best avoided.
- *Avoiding taking actions on behalf of clients that would be better undertaken by the clients themselves*: The norm in counselling is to help clients do things for themselves that they find challenging or have previously found impossible. Counsellors will usually avoid 'rescuing' clients from the consequences of their actions or the circumstances of their lives in order to create an opportunity to build client control. It is usually the exception that counsellors will cross boundaries into clients' areas of responsibility in order to intervene to protect them or others from serious harm or because they are legally required to do so.

There are exceptional circumstances when it may not be possible or desirable to maintain a firm boundary between counsellors' and clients' responsibilities, for example when clients are dependent on counsellors because their autonomy is substantially reduced by severe distress, illness, disability, intoxication or other causes. The aim in such situations would be to manage the boundaries in ways that would build on a client's capacity to act autonomously. Exceptionally there are ethical reasons for overriding a client's autonomous wishes to protect themself or others from serious harm. Sometimes the law will intervene and overrule a counsellor's professional ethics by requiring actions regardless of a client's wishes.

Nonetheless, the principle of respect for client autonomy requires paying carefully maintained attention to what are properly a counsellor's and client's responsibilities. This boundary between counsellor and client is most easily maintained when the latter enters counselling on a voluntary basis.

Stressing the Voluntary Nature of Counselling

It is a basic principle that counselling is a voluntary activity for the client. In most circumstances this is clearly the case: the client has sought out a counsellor as a matter of personal choice rather than feeling obliged to receive counselling or having been sent for counselling as an alternative to something worse (e.g. disciplinary action).

However, counsellors working in organizational settings report that there are situations where clients may be seeking counselling because they have been compelled to do so by someone else. For example, employee counsellors may have someone sent to them as an alternative to disciplinary procedures or as part of a disciplinary procedure. Counsellors in education also experience having clients sent to them, usually to resolve troublesome behaviour, but sometimes because a member of staff has recognized that a student is deeply distressed and needs help. Some people will seek counselling in all kinds of settings because they feel compelled to do so by partners, friends or their family. Usually the person sending the client is doing so out of a commitment to help and wants to act constructively. However, their action poses a number of difficulties for the counsellor. First, it challenges a client's ability to exercise choice about whether to participate in counselling. Second, there may be predetermined expectations about what the outcome of the counselling will be, and these are not necessarily those of the client. This may not be too much of a problem if the aim is to reduce distress, as the client is likely to share this aim. However, expectations about changes in the client's behaviour are likely to prove much more problematic.

Carl is sent to see a school counsellor to stop what his teacher sees as disruptive behaviour. During the counselling it emerges that Carl feels misunderstood and picked on by his teacher. He wants to find ways of expressing his views more effectively rather than becoming more compliant.

Any attempt by the counsellor to impose the teacher's views on Carl would clearly be in breach of the spirit of the voluntary nature of counselling and indicate a lack of respect for client autonomy.

A parallel situation also occurs with adults. Sometimes adults are sent to counsellors by employers as an alternative to disciplinary procedures. Again, this is usually done out of compassion for the client.

Joan is sent to an employee counsellor to help her reduce her lateness at starting work and her unexplained absences. The human resource manager who sent her suspects that she has relationship problems at home and has chosen this course of action rather than dismissing her as she is unlikely to be re-employed by anyone else.

Client autonomy

Beth has been sent by her employers to counselling. She doesn't want counselling – just the cause of her problems to stop. What should her counsellor do to respect her right to self-government?

There is considerable potential for confusion over client autonomy and the counsellor's role in these circumstances. What if Joan, unknown to the human resource manager, has been preparing to establish her own small business and this is why she is both absent and reluctant to offer an explanation? What if the human resource manager is right about the relationship **problems** causing the absence but Joan is happy to use these as an excuse and wants to go to counselling as a means of postponing the day of reckoning? In both these situations the counsellor may feel caught between the client's wishes and those of the human resource manager. Certainly, the counselling is unlikely to be effective because the client is not committed to the process; rather, she is using mere attendance as a shield against a less-liked alternative. This situation can be avoided by better management systems which would establish a clearer differentiation between disciplinary and counselling procedures.

It sometimes happens that a counsellor is not in a position to influence others in ways that prevent a client being 'sent'. For instance, a client may attend in compliance with a partner's wishes or under threat of someone else doing something that the client wants to prevent. The classic example would be someone accepting a detoxification from alcohol or drugs programme, which includes counselling, as an alternative to a custodial sentence or imprisonment. Can there be such a thing as a voluntary client who is under threat of imprisonment? This is one of many situations in which a counsellor cannot assume that it is the client's, rather than someone else's, wish that they receive counselling. It is good practice for counsellors to help clients establish their options, including not proceeding with the counselling. This may be a very quick process or may involve several sessions of 'pre-counselling' before a client is clear about whether they wish to proceed.

The ethical emphasis on consent as essential to respect for individual autonomy is paralleled by the law. Legally, adults in the UK (i.e. 18 years old and over) are entitled to give their consent or refuse any form of treatment unless the High Court has made a declaration of lawfulness to impose or withhold treatment. Young people aged 16–18 years old are also entitled to consent to or refuse any treatment, although a refusal to accept life-saving treatment can be overruled by the High Court (see the Family Law Reform Act 1969 s. 8(1) and the Age of Legal Capacity (Scotland) Act 1991). Below 16 years old, in accordance with the principles set by the House of Lords in *Gillick v West Norfolk* and *Wisbech Health Authority and Another* [1986]1 AC 112, a 'Gillick competent' young person of sufficient maturity, understanding and intelligence may give valid informed consent for treatment.

If a 'Gillick competent' young person refuses treatment, then their wishes should normally be respected, but if there is a need for treatment and parents (or others) who hold parental responsibility for the young person disagree with their child's decision or with each other, they can go to court and ask for a Specific Issue Order. If the young person is refusing treatment and the matter is serious, they can also apply to the High Court to resolve the issue. Assessing whether someone is of sufficient understanding and intelligence is a matter for an appropriately qualified service provider. For a young person to be competent (in terms of the Gillick case) to make a decision, factors to consider include:

- the age, maturity and understanding of the child;
- the information provided for the child;
- the nature of the decision to be made;
- the seriousness of the decision;
- the consequences of consent or refusal;
- the young person's ability to understand the wider context of the decision to be made.

In Scotland, in making any major decision about a child, a person with parental responsibility shall have regard to the views of the child concerned, and 'a child of twelve years of age or more shall be presumed to be of sufficient age and maturity to form a view' (s. 6 Children (Scotland) Act 1995). However, the ability of the child to express a view is not the same as allowing the child to make an informed decision, which requires 'Gillick competence'.

In both England and Scotland, the consent of a person with parental responsibility is required if the child is not 'Gillick competent' to make a decision. The consent of one person who has parental responsibility is sufficient. If more than one person has parental responsibility and they cannot agree on an important issue concerning their child, they can ask the family court to make an order where necessary. For further information about the law that is useful in working with children and young people, see Mitchels and Bond (2011) *Legal Issues across Counselling and Psychotherapy Settings*.

Failing to have obtained consent before offering counselling can lead to legal action for the civil wrongs (i.e. torts) of assault or, more likely in counselling, false imprisonment (misleadingly named, and better thought of as wrongful restraint). Legal aspects of informed consent are also considered in the context of suicide and confidentiality (see Chapters 7 and 10).

Encouraging Clients to Select Counsellors Who Meet Their Needs

The rapid growth of counselling means that there are increasing opportunities for clients to exercise personal choice as regards counsellors. For some clients this choice will centre on gender, or on the cultural and ethnic background of the counsellor. Often a client will be looking for someone with a similar background, but this is not necessarily the case.

A counselling service was being established for a large number of female refugees from a central African country. Counsellors were appointed from the same ethnic and cultural background in order to minimize the cultural barriers to potential clients. However, the service was little used until a white English woman was appointed. She discovered that potential clients were deterred by worries about confidentiality, and the possibility of details of their whereabouts or circumstances leaking back to their country of origin, with a potentially adverse impact on family members still living in a war zone.

This is one of the clearest examples of the dangers of making assumptions about who will be an acceptable counsellor for other people. The risk of getting this wrong is greatest when working across social differences. The best way of avoiding such mistakes is to be professionally curious, asking questions sensitively and listening carefully to the answers (see Chapter 12).

Increasingly, potential clients are being encouraged to 'shop around' in order to find the right type of therapy for them and the best available person to be their counsellor. Experience suggests that someone looking for a counsellor will have a number of issues to consider.

1. Being clear about what sort of help you want and the associated costs and potential benefits
    - What do you hope to get out of counselling – why are you seeking it? How could counselling successfully help you? In what ways could it fail you or make your situation worse? Are you looking to change things, or simply understand them better?
    - Do you want short- or long-term help? How much can you afford?
    - What type of therapy or therapist would suit you?
2. Finding a counsellor or therapist
    - Personal recommendations by someone who knows you well and whose judgment you trust are a good starting point. It helps if the person making the recommendation has used the service or has professional knowledge of others being helped by the recommended counsellor.
    - Consult directories provided by major national professional bodies such as the BACP, BPS, COSCA, IACP or UKCP.
    - Contact organizations specializing in the type of issue for which you want counselling to see if they can provide counselling or put you in touch with a recommended local counsellor. Good starting points are MIND or RELATE.
3. Choosing a counsellor or therapist

    Where possible contact two or three therapists before making a choice and ask them the following:
    - What qualifications do they have, and what sort of training was required to get these?
    - What experience have they in general and with the type of issues you want help with? What have been the outcomes for their clients?
    - Are they registered on either a statutory or **accredited voluntary register**, such as one accredited by the PSA? (Registration increases the **accountability** of the practitioner and can be viewed as a kite mark for the quality of service provided.)
    - Are they members of any professional organizations? Avoid counsellors and therapists who do not belong to reputable professional bodies or get around the question by saying 'I follow the ethical requirements of …'. If in doubt check with the professional body concerned online or by contacting their directory. Counsellors who are incompetent or exploitative tend to avoid such professional organizations or form small groups of like-minded people.
4. Rely on your instincts
    - If you don't like the way a therapist communicates with you, feel uneasy about whose needs are going to be met, or mistrust the counsellor for any

reason, do NOT go to them. You need to feel able to share private feelings and experiences freely with this person and to be confident that they will respect you as a person. Therapy is for your benefit as the client and not the other way round.

- If you have any concerns about the way your counsellor is working with you, discuss these with them at the earliest opportunity.
- One of the advantages of choosing a counsellor from a reputable professional organization is that you can consult this organization if you have any concerns that your counsellor is acting unprofessionally.
- If you conclude that your counsellor is acting unprofessionally, stop seeing them and report your concerns to their professional body.

Many counsellors also offer a trial session without obligation to either party to continue the counselling. This practice is a further demonstration of respect for client autonomy.

Providing Pre-counselling Information

A client's choice of counsellor can often be greatly assisted by the provision of information about the basis on which counselling is being provided. Such information might well provide:

- relevant background information about the counsellor(s);
- a brief definition or description of their counselling;
- a summary of what the client can expect of the counsellor;
- the client's responsibilities as regards receiving counselling;
- privacy policy – how any records concerning the client will be compiled and stored and how any communication about the client will be managed;
- any complaints procedure;
- arrangements for the payment of any fees.

Written and online mechanisms for pre-therapy communications with clients are critically important. Some are beautifully presented with colour graphics and photographs and include statements from former clients. The quality of presentation is primarily a marketing matter about how to communicate with potential clients effectively. Respect for client autonomy is communicated by the content and the degree to which a counsellor has anticipated the issues that concern potential clients.

One of the issues confronting anyone writing information for members of the public or clients about a counselling service is what to say about confidentiality. It is advisable to avoid statements like 'Counselling is totally confidential' because this arguably misrepresents the ethics of counselling and certainly the law (see Chapter 10). It is better to state simply that counselling is confidential, subject to the requirements of the law. If there are known circumstances in which confidentiality cannot be guaranteed these should be mentioned, or if the circumstances have only a remote possibility of arising, potential clients could be encouraged to raise any issues about confidentiality with their counsellor. This might involve making a statement like:

> Counsellors understand that confidentiality can be very important to anyone seeking counselling. If you would like further information about the level of confidentiality we offer or any other matter, please ask the counsellor about it at the beginning of the session.

The basic principle is that all clients should know the terms on which they are being offered confidentiality. In particular, they should know all the circumstances in which confidentiality is *not* possible. Respect for client autonomy requires that clients are adequately informed about any limits to confidentiality and have consented to receiving counselling on this basis. This is a legal requirement for the **processing** of any personally identifiable information concerning clients and should contain the following information (Mitchels and Bond, 2021):

- Contact details.
- The types of personal data you process.
- Lawful basis for processing personal data.
- How you process personal data.
- How long you will be keeping their data.
- Data subject rights.

It is ethically better to produce information that is specific to the counselling being provided, and in a style appropriate to the client group. This information may be provided in pre-counselling leaflets or on a website. Sometimes this will require providing information in languages other than English and additionally ensuring that information is available to people with disabilities (e.g. in Braille). It may also require imaginative use of drawings for clients who are unable to read or the opportunity for preliminary pre-counselling discussions with a receptionist or counsellor about the suitability of counselling.

Clear Contracting

Counselling is not unique in attaching considerable importance to client autonomy. There is also an increasing emphasis on autonomy in professions that have sometimes been considered paternalistic in their concern to do good for someone. Nowhere is this change more evident than in medicine. Reiter-Theil et al. (1991) observed that 'Derived from the principle of *respect for autonomy*, informed consent has become one of the predominant rules discussed in medical ethics since the 1970s.'

Informed consent is someone's agreement to treatment after having understood:

- the procedures or methods to be used;
- any risks and benefits;
- being informed of relevant alternatives.

It must be guaranteed that a client consented without coercion or manipulation and that they are able to make a rational decision based on the information provided. However, consent is the absolute minimum standard of practice in counselling. It is more appropriate to situations where a person has something done to them, rather than as in counselling where the client is an active participant. Most ethical guidelines for counsellors require a higher standard of actively engaging clients in the contracting process. All the major professional bodies in the UK, and most internationally, require that counsellors are responsible for establishing clear and explicit contracts with clients at the start of the relationship. The BACP *Ethical Framework* is typical in linking contracting to respect for client autonomy and the importance of building an appropriate relationship. On this it states:

> We will give careful consideration to how we reach agreement with clients and will contract with them about the terms on which our services will be provided. Attention will be given to:
>
> - reaching an agreement or contract that takes account of each client's expressed needs and choices so far as possible
> - communicating terms and conditions of the agreement or contract in ways easily understood by the client and appropriate to their context
> - stating clearly how a client's confidentiality and privacy will be protected and any circumstances in which confidential or private information will be communicated to others
> - providing the client with a record or easy access to a record of what has been agreed
> - keeping a record of what has been agreed and of any changes or clarifications when they occur
> - being watchful for any potential contractual incompatibilities between agreements with our clients and any other contractual agreements applicable to the work being undertaken and proactively strive to avoid these wherever possible or promptly alert the people with the power or responsibility to resolve these contradictions. (BACP, 2018a: 17)

Two issues are frequently raised by counsellors: whether the contract can be based on a spoken rather than a written agreement and how to manage situations where the client is more concerned to get started with the counselling than to discuss contractual arrangements. There are no ethical or legal reasons which require that the therapeutic contract should be in writing, although it is now generally considered helpful to ensure that the client fully understands the terms on which counselling is being offered. The contract may serve other purposes in addition to demonstrating respect for client autonomy. It can be a method of reinforcing the agreed therapeutic goals or purpose of the counselling, as well as being a reference point for review at stages in the counselling process. It may also establish a legally enforceable agreement between counsellor and client.

Whenever a client is paying fees or, albeit rarely and best avoided, offering a service in lieu of fees, for example gardening or decorating, any agreement between counsellor and client is legally enforceable. It is also arguable in law that a therapeutic contract may be held to exist and be enforceable in some circumstances when counselling is provided to the client free of charge. A written record of the agreement in the form of a signed statement, contemporaneous record in the case notes, or a letter sent to the client confirming what has been agreed, reduces the risk of contradictory memories arising later. An oral contract is legally enforceable but is much more vulnerable to being contradicted subsequently in any legal dispute or professional complaints procedure.

The ethical emphasis on clear contracting at the start of counselling is sometimes at odds with the practical experience of working with clients. Some will be committed to starting counselling as quickly as possible, either because of their level of distress or the urgency of the issue that is concerning them. In these circumstances, it can be difficult to enter into meaningful negotiations over a contract and the act of doing so may seem disrespectful of the client's obvious wish to get on with the counselling. This is one of the situations which can be eased by providing pre-counselling information and simply checking with the client whether they have read this and are willing to proceed on that basis. The contractual arrangements can be reviewed once this initial urgency has subsided.

Contracting

Michael wants to start his counselling immediately. How should the counsellor respond? How can she respect his wishes whilst also making sure he understands what is involved and what he is committing himself to? What is bad practice? What is good practice?

- Name, address.
- Contact details (and any limitations).
- Fee structure and policy (hourly rate, charges for missed sessions, fee for time spent on phone calls, writing reports, action on non-payment etc.).
- Frequency and duration of sessions (will dates and times be fixed and regular or will each appointment be negotiated?).
- Likely duration of therapy (e.g. is it time-limited or open-ended, and if open-ended, are estimated duration and/or regular reviews necessary for funding or other purposes?).
- Policy for non-attendance (e.g. will therapy be withdrawn for non-attendance without a reasonable excuse or explanation?).
- Holidays.
- Cancellation of sessions by therapist or client.
- Terminating therapy (deciding when and how to end therapy).
- Contact between sessions (when and where can the client call the therapist?).
- Confidentiality issues (e.g. the legal limits of confidentiality. Does the client consent to share information? In what circumstances? Referral procedures and client instructions and consents).
- Any information and consents relevant for possible referrals.
- Record keeping (e.g. how long will records be kept?).
- Client right of access to records.
- Use of records for supervision, research, audit and so on.
- Relevant data protection issues and any explicit consents required for sensitive personal data.
- Tape and other recordings of sessions (ownership, access, potential uses and retention).
- Counsellor's professional memberships, code of ethics, insurance and information about complaints procedures.

Case history and referral information may be sought and specific aspects can be reflected in the contract if this is appropriate, or for the safety of the client or others:

- Relevant case history.
- General practitioner details.
- Other professionals' reports.
- Other professionals' agencies, family or friends to be contacted with the client's consent if therapeutically necessary or appropriate to support the client or for the safety of the client or others.

FIGURE 6.1 *Checklist for items to consider including in a contract (Mitchels and Bond, 2010)*

It is generally considered good practice to periodically review the contractual relationship with a client. BACP's *Ethical Framework* states that 'We will periodically review each client's progress and, when practicable, seek our client's views on how we are working together' (2018a: 17). These reviews will probably concentrate on the therapeutic aims and achievements of the counselling but might well also include clarification of expectations over confidentiality or practical arrangements. The therapeutic and legal basis of the relationship may be changed by such reviews.

Figure 6.1 provides an overview of the key issues that are usually included within a written counselling contract for face-to-face counselling. Additional issues to be considered for online counselling can be found within Chapter 11 and Example 3 in Chapter 17.

Respecting Clients' Values, Beliefs and Choice of Action

One of the major challenges in respecting client autonomy is offering respect to values and beliefs which may be quite different from one's own or considered unacceptable within one's own social or cultural group. (The challenges of counselling across social **diversity** are considered more fully in Chapter 12.) How far ought a counsellor go to respect their client's values when these are substantially different from their own? What if the client's values, beliefs or choice of actions conflict with the counsellor's autonomous views?

Relationship between Counsellor and Client Autonomy

The optimum standard in counselling is that both the counsellor and client are working together as a deliberate and autonomous choice. This is most likely to happen when they share important personal values; however, this is not essential. Counselling often takes place where there are differences in values, but a counsellor's personal values favour respect for their clients' values, beliefs and choices and a commitment to working within these. In reality, it is probably most often the case that counsellors and clients work together satisfactorily where their personal values are compatible rather than identical. The onus is on counsellors to provide clients with sufficient space to work within their own value system, with a counsellor's own value system validating this relationship and avoiding the imposition of that counsellor's own personal values. Without a counsellor's commitment to respecting a client's values and capacity for self-determination, their relationship will lack integrity. Integrity requires that both counsellor and client are acting autonomously.

However, such a relationship is a high standard to maintain and it is not always easy to do so. What should a counsellor do when they find themself working with a client whose personal values are so antagonistic to their own that both the integrity of the counselling relationship and the counsellor's own personal integrity are threatened?

Mark is a committed pacifist for religious and personal reasons. He has counselled soldiers recovering from post-traumatic stress disorder who are returning to civilian life. Does respect for a client's values, beliefs and capacity for self-determination mean that he should also be willing to counsel soldiers wishing to return to active military service?

Mark's dilemma is encountered in many forms. To what extent does respect for client autonomy require that counsellors work with clients who choose to act in ways which conflict with a counsellor's deeply held views?

There is often a baseline to good practice which is respectful of client autonomy while allowing a counsellor to maintain a conscientiously held moral position. The general expectation is that a counsellor is willing to work with a wide range of people with values that differ from their own. Counsellors ought not to refuse to work with clients because of differences in values alone. Any valid barriers to taking on clients ought not to be about values but could include issues of competence, a counsellor's acceptability to a client, and a counsellor's sense of safety from physical or sustained psychological attack. Even in situations of significant clashes of values between counsellor and client, a counsellor ought to be willing to respect the humanity of their client sufficiently to find them a more appropriate counselling service.

Pro-life counselling

Some counsellors hold strong personal views against abortion and treat this as a matter of conscience. Such counsellors may be working in settings where they see clients about a wide range of **issues** so that the question of abortion may be raised only infrequently. Alternatively, they may be working in one of the pro-life organizations as a counsellor with the explicit aim of providing alternatives to abortion. What should a counsellor do if a client decides she wants an abortion? It is incompatible with even a minimal level of respect for client autonomy merely to say 'I disagree with your choice and can do no more. Come and see me again if you change your mind.' The minimum level of respect is to give the client sufficient information to enable her to implement her choice. Ideally, the counsellor would actively enable a referral to someone who could be more supportive of that client's autonomous choices.

Christian counselling

Many counselling services that identify themselves with the Christian counselling movement resolve the issue of protecting the integrity of their services by being explicit about their religious orientation. They may explicitly state that they work 'according to biblical assumptions, aims and methods practised within a framework of Christian commitment, insight and values'. Where these services are provided to like-minded people, the issue of respect for client autonomy is neutralized. However, when these services are provided to the general public, there is a considerable clash between the ethics and values of counselling incorporating a narrowly defined religious agenda and those working within the ethical principles advocated in this book. The principle of autonomy would require a counsellor to work with respect for any religious beliefs of their clients, whether that client identified with Christian or other religious faiths or had no religious affiliations. This would be difficult for anyone who held any form of fundamentalist belief to achieve.

When cases have been heard in relationship to the ethics of the American Counseling Association (ACA) and the British Association of Counselling and Psychotherapy (BACP), it has been held that it is unacceptable to refuse services to people in same-sex relationships because the counsellor takes a conservative Christian view and believes such relationships are wrong.

The type of Christian counselling just described should not be confused with counselling which is provided by someone who has Christian beliefs but respects a client's right to hold different religious beliefs or no beliefs at all. There is a long-established tradition of pastoral counselling which is based on respect for a client's autonomy over religious beliefs (Hiltner, 1949; Wise, 1951; Foskett and Lyall, 1988; Lynch, 2002). The place of faith, spirituality and prayer, for example, is ably discussed and explored with sensitivity by Gubi (2008, 2015, 2017).

Similar issues arise in other faith traditions. Faith is a major resource in times of crisis for many people that builds resilience in the face of extreme losses and trauma or other personally challenging circumstances. Clients' faith, or lack of faith, is core to their identity and an important point of reference in how they exercise their autonomy. The challenge for counsellors working within an ethic of respect for client autonomy and a commitment to respecting social diversity is how to find ways of valuing this aspect of their clients' lives when their beliefs may be very different from their own.

Racist or sexist clients

It is ethically consistent with the core values of counselling of respect, integrity and impartiality that counsellors should strive to provide counselling services on the basis of equality of opportunity for users of the service. A deliberately racist or sexist counsellor could not subscribe to counselling values with personal integrity. This raises the question 'How should a counsellor respond to a client who does not share these values?' It is not uncommon for counsellors to seek **guidance** from counsellors who have been deeply troubled by the racism and sexism of some clients.

Rachel is conscientious in attempting to establish relationships with her clients that have the qualities of integrity, impartiality and respect. Tom, the client, is deeply committed to views that are intolerant and often exploitative of people with different ethnic origins from his own, and these are the basis of his chosen courses of action. How should Rachel respond?

Most counsellors accept that there can be no automatic duty placed on a counsellor to challenge a client's views. Counselling needs to be provided in ways that permit clients to express views which differ considerably from those of the counsellor. Respect for a client's right to express anti-social views and negative feelings towards others has always been an important part of respect for a client's capacity for self-determination. It is also part of the therapeutic process, in which such feelings sometimes change. Therefore, the counselling relationship is not an appropriate place to campaign for greater social tolerance. However, on occasions this effect may be achieved by the resolution of areas of personal pain which fuel intolerance. But this analysis does not resolve Rachel's dilemma. She is faced with a client whose personal values are so different from her own that she no longer feels able to offer respect for his capacity for self-determination without sacrificing her personal integrity. In her view, the situation is not resolved by maintaining clear boundaries between her own value system and those of her client. In these circumstances it seems appropriate to consider discussing the conflict of personal values with the client directly.

It is only once the issue has been discussed openly between the counsellor and client that each of them will be in a position to decide whether it is desirable to continue counselling together. How to raise the subject and the timing of the discussion may need to be considered in counselling supervision. However, to continue without raising the subject is open to objections from both the counsellor's and client's viewpoints. It is not possible to conscientiously help someone to live their life according to their own values when a counsellor strongly disapproves of those values. Equally, a client may have valid moral grounds for objecting to being counselled by someone who has kept disapproval of their values secret from them. This could be viewed as covertly undermining client autonomy. The integrity of the relationship requires finding a basis on which both counsellor and client can proceed by respecting each other's autonomy. Alternatively, it may be better to discontinue counselling and for the counsellor to assist the client in finding an alternative source of help if this is requested. Issues of this degree of difficulty are best discussed in counselling supervision or with another experienced counsellor before deciding how to respond to a client. The example given above is about racism but could equally have been about prejudices based on gender, disability, sexuality, class, religion or age. Ethically, it is important that a counsellor responds to this dilemma in a way that is both consistent with the counselling model being used and respectful of the client's choice of outcome. To act otherwise is to move outside the ethical boundaries of relationships in counselling. For example, persuasion and manipulation to seek to change someone's point of view, even for what are widely held to be socially desirable ends, are intrusions into an area of responsibility which is properly the client's.

Social Justice in Context

The provision of counselling has, over the years, developed so that it can now be found in a range of settings and contexts, for example schools, colleges, universities, third sector, health and social care settings, independent practice and online. Alongside this, the diversity of communities for whom counselling may be a positive choice through which to explore emotional distress has increased also. Counselling that pays attention to the principles of social justice (e.g. equality, respect, autonomy, free choice) must ensure that it does this in an active way. As explored in other chapters of this book, working in the context of social justice demands action to attend to social injustice. Reflecting on similarities and differences between values and life experiences of counsellors and their clients, and how they can be positively engaged with, is arguably a cultural and social imperative.

At times, some counsellors may feel frustration with the need to respect their clients' responsibility for the outcome of the counselling. One way some counsellors have found of resolving this ethically has been to accept the constraints on their range of personal responses when in a counselling role with particular clients. However, independent of counselling, they will offer workshops, lectures, or write or campaign to try to change attitudes. There is a tradition within counselling which goes back to Frank Parsons (1854–1908), the probable originator of the term 'counselling', and his campaigns on behalf of the urban poor in Boston during the early 1900s, which combined counselling with social and political action. In the UK, this tradition has continued in some areas of the country and within movements to empower disadvantaged people, particularly women and gay or lesbian people. Equally, there has been a tradition which is less activist and more politically quietist. It seems to us that both traditions are valid here. They present potential clients with a range of choices between a variety of counsellors with different values and personal views about how best to implement those values.

Pause for Reflection

Consider the issues that might present in counselling that you would find most difficult to work with. What are these issues, do you have a sense of what informs your own position, and how might you manage that conflict ethically?

Limitations to Respect for Autonomy

What is the limit of respect for individual autonomy? Two of the major ethical systems that have influenced western society accept that there is a limit to the principle of autonomy. The ethical system founded by Immanuel Kant which prioritizes autonomy over ethical issues and views people as ends in themselves recognizes that there is a point where one person's right to autonomy may conflict with another's. Similarly, John Stuart Mill (1806–1873), an exponent of utilitarianism, an ethic committed to achieving the 'greatest happiness of the greatest number', argued strongly for the importance of respecting another's autonomy. However, he also imposed restrictions. The person whose autonomy is respected should possess a fairly basic level of maturity and therefore be capable of taking responsibility for their own autonomous actions. As a philosopher, Mill was primarily concerned with the rationality of people and this is reflected in his test for an adequate level of maturity, which he defined as 'a capability of being improved by free and equal discussion' (Mill, 1859: 15). These two restrictions recur as issues in counselling.

To access the online resources accompanying this chapter, please visit: https://study.sagepub.com/reevesandbond

7

Suicide and Refusing to Accept Life-saving Treatment

Chapter Overview

Suicidal intent is one of the most challenging ethical issues faced by counsellors. This chapter considers the choice between respecting client **autonomy** and the commitment to do good by acting to preserve a client's life, and some of the criteria that ought to be taken into account. Recommendations from NICE about a person-centred assessment strategy are considered. Different motivations for **suicide** are distinguished for ethical analysis. The chapter concludes with the refusal to accept **life-saving treatment**.

Key words

suicidal intent, suicide, self-harm, assessment, treatment, self-administered **euthanasia**, refusal to consent, death

Some of the situations which counsellors encounter cause great anxiety. Working with clients who are seriously intent on **suicide** must be one of the most anxiety provoking because of the sense of imminent death, which makes any decisions and actions irreversible. The choice between life and death is a stark one. At a time when a counsellor's therapeutic skills are being considerably tested, there are also major ethical **issues** to consider. We are faced with a choice between respecting client **autonomy** or seeking to preserve life, either because this is considered to be a fundamental ethical principle or because it is thought to be in the client's best interests. Unfortunately, it is an issue that appears to be surrounded with misunderstanding about the ethical and legal parameters that apply here. It is probable that many counsellors and professional agencies will want to review their existing practice in light of recent clarifications of the **law** as applied by the English legal system.

The Suicidal Client

Clients who are seriously intent on suicide present counsellors with an acute ethical dilemma. The choice is between respecting client autonomy or intervening in the interest of preserving life. Counsellors remain divided about how best to resolve this ethical dilemma. One view takes the primacy of life as an ethical cornerstone. This is founded on the belief that life is the most valuable thing we possess: life is so obviously good that it requires no theoretical argument to justify its position as a primary value. It is asserted that the sanctity of life is self-evident, especially one's own life. The act of questioning its value is therefore in itself symptomatic of crisis, illness or abnormality. From this moral perspective it is easy to justify acting to prevent someone taking their own life. The force of this justification would even override a client's autonomous wishes in order to compel them to accept treatment or confinement without the opportunity to kill themself. The experience of many mental health professionals appears to match this particular analysis. They report that suicidal feelings are often short-lived and transitory. If someone can be protected from acting on these feelings, then the will to live often returns and the **problems** which have caused this person to become suicidal can be tackled. Reeves offers an in-depth discussion of working with clients at risk of suicide (Reeves, 2010, 2015).

There is an alternative point of view that the number of people who continue to die through suicide challenges any claim to the self-evident sanctity of life. Occasions arise when the desire to preserve life may be overridden by a preference for death. From this perspective, suicide is the ultimate expression of someone's choice of how to live or die. It follows that counsellors ought to **respect** clients' right of choice over their suicide in the same way as they would over other matters. R.D. Laing (1967) also believed that suicide was the ultimate right of any individual. Szasz (1986) has argued that any attempt at coercive methods to prevent suicide contradicts the concept of individuals as moral agents, who are ultimately responsible for their own actions. Some counsellors take this view and apply it consistently to all situations involving suicide. This stance is particularly attractive if, like Laing and Szasz, a counsellor disagrees with the medicalization of mental illness and does not accept that behaviour which others have defined as mental illness erodes an individual's moral **responsibility** for their own actions.

It is also a point of view which appeals to therapists working with the large number of people who go through the motions of attempting suicide but appear to have no real intention of killing themselves. Known as 'parasuicide', this is primarily a cry for help. Part of a counsellor's role is to encourage clients to communicate what is wanted more directly, and therefore to act with a greater sense of control over their autonomy. To rush into a course of action designed to prevent suicide would be counter-therapeutic. It might reinforce any manipulative component in the parasuicide rather than reinforce clients' ability to act more straightforwardly in the quest to resolve their problems.

The proponents of each of these views can argue that their opinions are founded on an ethical analysis and within a constructive framework which enhance therapeutic work with significant numbers of the suicidal. How should a counsellor choose between them? An analysis of the situations in which counsellors encounter clients who are contemplating suicide suggests that the appropriate response ought to be varied according to each client's circumstances. The **law** in many jurisdictions has not left matters so open-ended, however. Different legal systems have tended to favour resolving the ethical dilemma in favour of one or other of the competing ethical principles. English law is no exception to this tendency, as will become apparent. This may provide some relief to those who find uncertainty in these circumstances almost too much to bear.

Suicide as self-administered euthanasia

Sally has terminal cancer and has been told by doctors that her illness is well advanced, with an increasing number of secondaries. She has announced to her family and her doctor that she does not wish to battle futilely against her imminent death. She would prefer to die at home at a time of her own choosing. Her family and doctor attempt to dissuade her or suggest alternative ways of providing good-quality terminal care, but Sally remains committed to her planned suicide and has discussed her plans with her counsellor over several months.

This is the kind of situation where there can be little doubt that the client is making a decision that is authentic, deliberate and clearheaded. She has sustained her point of view over a period of time and is acting under her own volition, not under the influence of others. It may be that the counsellor will want to check that the client is aware of alternative ways of receiving care during a terminal illness, and that her aims would not be better met by home nursing, or the use of a living will in which the client sets out how she wishes to be cared for medically, or going into a hospice. Even if the client is unaware of any of these, or feels that they are inadequate to enable her to take control of her dying, there are unlikely to be grounds for the counsellor to intervene to attempt to prevent her suicide (although it would be illegal for the counsellor to actively assist a person to end their own life). Heyd and Bloch (1991) express the view that although doctors will find it psychologically and legally difficult to co-operate actively in such a suicide, no psychiatrist would consider the forced hospitalization of such a person. Under current mental health legislation that applies in England and Wales, the Mental Health Act 2007, there is no provision for compulsory assessment or treatment merely because someone is suicidal. It is well established in English law that adults have the right to refuse treatment even if to do so would result in their own death. This means that, even if a counsellor wanted to intervene, there would be very little that could be imposed to override a client's intent.

Counselling a client with suicidal intent

Clare has recently received some medical test results. Her diagnosis is bad news. She has a disease that will eventually destroy her quality of life and kill her. How should her counsellor respond, particularly when she talks about ending her life? What are the most important issues to consider?

The counsellor may experience further dilemmas. What if the family seek the counsellor's support in trying to persuade Sally out of self-administered **euthanasia**? This is a situation where the counsellor needs to consider the nature of the **contract** with the client and, assuming that this contract is with Sally, may have to explain tactfully that her primary responsibility is to Sally, who retains control of the outcome of the counselling. If the family feel unable to communicate their feelings about Sally's proposed actions directly to her, then they may wish to use another counsellor to facilitate such a discussion. For Sally's counsellor to undertake an additional role on behalf of the family could raise all the problems of conflicting loyalties, particularly as there is a substantial difference of view between them.

An alternative possibility is that the counsellor feels strongly supportive of Sally's decision to take control of her own dying. How far should she go in offering emotional encouragement or active support? Legally there are definite limits to how far a counsellor can go without risking prosecution. Unlike Dutch or Swiss law, there is no provision for doctors or anyone else to assist someone to end their own life. The legalization of euthanasia is discussed periodically, but it seems unlikely that this will happen soon. Until there is a change in the law, it is a criminal offence to assist someone to kill themselves. Although the Suicide Act 1961 stopped attempted suicide and suicide from being a criminal offence, it also created a new offence. Section 2 states:

> A person who aids, abets, counsels or procures the suicide of another or an attempt by another to commit suicide, shall be liable on conviction on indictment to imprisonment for a term not exceeding fourteen years.

To 'counsel' in this legal context means to conspire, advise or knowingly give assistance, all of which are not activities usually encompassed within counselling. Although the Mental Capacity Act 2005 has strengthened the rights of adults to consent to and refuse treatment (see later in this chapter), this legislation explicitly excludes consent to assisted suicide, which remains a criminal offence by the person who offers assistance.

Suicide as an Escape from Problems and Emotional Pain

Another example describes the kind of situation which most counsellors encounter fairly frequently.

Brian is over-burdened by financial problems and social isolation following the ending of a long-standing relationship. He is becoming increasingly depressed and is talking about suicide as a way out of his problems and to escape the emotional pain he is experiencing.

In this example Brian's suicide is not an alternative to an imminent and inevitable death, but represents a substantial foreshortening of his lifespan. There is also an element of doubt about whether his choice is authentic, deliberate, clear-headed and rational, or whether he is acting irrationally, impulsively and on the basis of a judgment distorted by extreme personal distress or the loss of a sense of reality. Our knowledge of how best to understand and help in such circumstances is becoming better informed by **research** (O'Connor, 2010) and professional **guidance** (BACP, 2020b) but is still far from complete. All mental health professionals are faced with complex judgments around the circumstances of a particular person. A key ethical dimension for counsellors in circumstances like these is the choice between respecting client autonomy and acting to prevent a client's self-destruction.

It is tempting with such a difficult ethical dilemma to turn to the law as a way of pre-empting the ethical choice. The fear that an ethical dilemma might turn into legal liability makes this a very natural reaction. Many turn to the law in the expectation that it will justify an intervention to preserve life and thus end the dilemma. In practice, the law does not provide such an instant solution. For most counsellors there is no clear-cut obligation to intervene on behalf of adults. English law is strongly weighted in favour of respecting individual autonomy, especially of adults. A subsidiary issue arises because a counsellor will not usually have the power to intervene directly. Any offer of treatment in addition to the counselling will require the services of a doctor, psychiatrist, psychiatric nurse, social worker or approved mental health professional. The ethical dilemma is eliminated where a client is willing to seek the help of these services on their own behalf. Many clients will appreciate their counsellor's clear suggestion that there are additional sources of help and that it would be appropriate to contact these. Some clients may request that the counsellor help them to make contact with the service, especially if they are depressed, which is the commonest reason for feeling suicidal. Many counsellors would feel ethically obliged to respond to a client's request for assistance in these circumstances, unless there are good grounds for thinking that this would be inappropriate.

David is a student teacher who has chosen to see a counsellor privately rather than see the university counsellor or the one attached to his doctor's practice. He has made this decision because he wants to protect the confidentiality of the counselling. However, his counsellor insists that he inform his GP or she will do so when he discloses that he is feeling suicidal. David refuses to do so because he does not want his emotional state to be recorded on his medical notes. He is concerned this might have negative implications for his medical assessment for suitability to practise.

A frequent reason for refusing medical assistance in these circumstances is a concern that once a GP is involved the information may be subsequently disclosed in medical reports for employers or **insurance** companies. It is not only counsellors who have issues around dual relationships and their consequences for service users. Some counselling services have lists of doctors and psychiatrists who will see people privately. Let us suppose that this client continues to reject all suggestions that he should seek psychiatric help. The counsellor points out that both her professional **codes** and her original agreement with him permit her to breach **confidentiality** when she considers that there is a serious risk of the client harming himself. He still refuses to allow her to do so. Many counsellors might consider that they are legally obliged to inform in these circumstances and that they will be protected from claims for breach of confidentiality if they do so. These are misunderstandings of the English legal system, which from Magna Carta onwards through a long series of medical cases has protected the adult citizen's right to refuse medical treatment.

The expectation that counsellors have a **duty of care** to protect clients from **suicidal intent** may be based on misapplications of US law. In most states, counsellors are required to breach confidentiality to report a client's suicidal intent. There is no equivalent requirement in the UK. Nor is there any legal protection against an action for breach of confidentiality in the above example. The counsellor could be liable for substantial damages for loss of earnings if the client's career were to be adversely affected by an inappropriate **disclosure**. Although there is no general duty to intervene, some special circumstances may create such a duty. For example, a counsellor working with patients receiving compulsory psychiatric treatment under the Mental Health Act 2007 may have an obligation to intervene under the terms of their contract of employment or other aspects of civil law. However, this obligation does not automatically transfer to counsellors who are working independently of the statutory mental health services.

In the case of adults, it is only when a counsellor has reasonable grounds for believing that a client is seriously at risk of attempting suicide *and* is suffering a treatable mental disorder (e.g. depression, schizophrenia) that it may be defensible to breach confidence in order to seek an assessment to determine whether that client should be compelled to receive compulsory treatment under the Mental Health Act. This Act explicitly excludes promiscuity and alcohol or drug dependency from its provisions for compulsory assessment or treatment orders. It is defensible to breach confidences where someone is being coerced into suicide in order to prevent a serious criminal offence. However, the current law urges considerable caution with regard to overriding an adult's refusal to permit a counsellor to breach confidentiality in order to protect an adult intent from causing harm to themself, even if the consequences might be fatal.

The law takes a robust view of adult autonomy and will generally protect it unless other people are being placed at risk by the intended behaviour (e.g. jumping into traffic on a public road). However, a counsellor is permitted to repeatedly offer additional assistance and to try to find a form of help that would be acceptable to the person concerned. Obtaining a client's consent for other forms of assistance is not only the best legal protection, but is also the best way of ensuring that client's collaboration in any subsequent treatment. The balance of **public interest** switches more strongly in favour of seeking assistance for someone aged 16–18 in order to avert a life-threatening situation. It is completely reversed in the case of young people of insufficient intelligence or understanding to be considered 'Gillick competent' (see later in this chapter, and Chapters 6 and 10). For young people there are provisions in children and young persons' legislation which provide alternatives to the use of mental health legislation. Further **advice** can be obtained from the relevant local children's services department, the NSPCC or MIND.

One of the consequences of this legal protection of adult autonomy is that it places greater ethical emphasis on counsellors being clear about the extent to which they feel competent to work with suicidal clients. A counsellor has a right to withdraw from counselling when they feel that counselling is beyond their **competence** and a client refuses additional assistance or referral. In reaching a decision about whether to work with a particular client or how best to do so, a counsellor may wish to consider the degree of suicidal risk. This is not only to the advantage of clients who are looking to a counsellor to help them overcome self-destructive feelings, but is also in the counsellor's self-interest in terms of having some control over the scale of the challenge they are taking on.

Pause for Reflection

What are your personal views in relation to suicide, and what things in your own life have shaped this perspective, for example experience of mental health crisis in yourself or someone close to you, faith or training. How might your views influence how you respond to suicidal crisis in your clients?

NICE guidelines (CG133, 2011) on working with people who **self-harm**, which includes suicidal intent, have adopted a person-centred approach that requires all health and social care workers to:

- aim to develop a trusting, supportive and engaging relationship with them;
- be aware of the **discrimination** and stigma sometimes associated with self-harm, both in the wider society and the health service, and adopt a non-judgmental approach;
- ensure that people are fully involved in decision making about their treatment and care;
- aim to foster people's autonomy and independence wherever possible;
- maintain the continuity of therapeutic relationships wherever possible;
- ensure that information about episodes of self-harm is communicated sensitively to other members of the team.

A comprehensive psychosocial assessment of needs is recommended for the longer-term management of self-harm, which should include:

- skills, strengths and assets;
- coping strategies;
- mental health problems or disorders;
- social circumstances and problems;
- psychosocial and occupational functioning, and vulnerabilities;
- recent and current life difficulties, including personal and financial problems;
- the need for psychological intervention, social care and support, occupational rehabilitation, and also drug treatment for any associated conditions;
- the needs of any dependent children.

The advice on the use of assessment tools and scales is unequivocal:

- Do not use risk assessment tools and scales to predict future suicide or repetition of self-harm.

Instead, the NICE guidelines (2011) recommend a more individualized assessment of the risk of any repetition of self-harm or suicide by agreeing with the person concerned the specific risks for them, taking into account:

- the methods and patterns of current or past self-harm;
- specific risk factors and protective factors (social, psychological, pharmacological, and motivational) that may increase or decrease the risks associated with self-harm;
- coping strategies that the person has used to either successfully limit or avert self-harm or to contain the impact of personal, social or other antecedents.

The assessment of suicidal intent often involves difficult decisions. It is in both the client's and counsellor's interests that the counsellor holds appropriate discussions with a counselling supervisor or experienced counsellor and, if necessary, seeks the opinions of professionals with relevant experience. The purpose of these consultations is to provide support for the counsellor, clarify the issues that require consideration, and provide any additional information not already known by the counsellor or client, especially about the kinds of help available from non-counselling services. Accurate and up-to-date information about these services and counselling helps to ensure that the client is in a position to make informed choices about the kind of help they want.

Any consultations by the counsellor with people outside the counselling relationship which are undertaken as part of the assessment stage should either be with the client's consent or undertaken in such a way that the client's identity is not disclosed. The assumption of respect for client autonomy carries with it the high **standards** of practice concerning confidentiality. These consultations are not an alternative to the client's making these enquiries for themself, which is the usual practice in counselling. It is highly desirable that wherever possible the client make their own enquiries as a means of taking control of their own destiny.

The process of assessing suicidal clients is often therapeutic to those who actively participate in the assessment procedure. Often what seems an overwhelming and ill-defined sense of hopelessness does change into a differentiated series of separate problems which can seem more manageable. Perhaps most importantly, the counsellor is giving the client permission to explore their suicidal feelings and discover what these really mean for them, with the possibility of finding alternative outcomes. The assessment process is often a time when clients have a sense of starting to deal with the issues which really concern them. This sense of a new start is often accompanied by a willingness to put suicidal intentions to one side for the time being in the hope of making changes to make life more rewarding. It is also appropriate to ensure that a client knows where to get help in an emergency (usually from their doctor, a hospital accident and emergency department or the Samaritans, depending on which is acceptable to that client), which can often be helpfully outlined in a collaboratively agreed crisis plan. Some excellent examples are available online, via the Papyrus UK website (www.papyrus-uk.org) and the Students Against Depression website (www.studentsagainstdepression.org).

For a counsellor, a systematic assessment procedure provides a means of resolving an ethical dilemma in a considered and conscientious way. Although it is not always possible to be infallible in this regard, at least the counsellor knows that they have done all that can reasonably be expected of them and has also maximized the likelihood of a client making an authentic and considered choice. Many counsellors working with suicidal clients would also assert the importance of not taking significant decisions without consultation with at least one other person. If a client does die through suicide, a counsellor may experience regret and concern that, perhaps, something more could have been done to prevent this. It is at times like these that it is useful to know that the decision was not taken on one's own. Consultations with a counselling supervisor, doctor or social worker are a simple way of helping to minimize the inevitable distress following some suicides. In practice, many clients will consent to these discussions if they can be reassured that they are adequately protected by confidentiality and that they will enhance the quality of the counselling they receive. In our experience, many clients view this way of working as evidence that counsellors are taking their needs seriously.

Refusing to Accept Life-saving Treatment

Suicide requires someone to take positive action that places their life in jeopardy. Counsellors may also encounter situations where someone is facing premature death as a result of their inaction. This may be someone who is refusing medical treatment for a treatable illness which, if untreated, will result in death. Counsellors working with people with eating disorders will be familiar with this situation. Some people with anorexic conditions will refuse all offers of treatment and eventually starve themselves to death. Not all refusals to eat to the point of becoming life-threatening are medically diagnosable. Some people will refuse to eat to draw attention to a particular cause (e.g. hunger strikers). Religious convictions may lead others to refuse certain **life-saving treatments**. The best known of these is the refusal of blood transfusions by Jehovah's Witnesses. In contrast to these considered refusals, some people are simply so disturbed or confused that they either fail to understand the significance of not accepting treatment or are incapable of co-operating with any treatment regime on a **voluntary** basis.

As with suicidal intent, the refusal of life-saving treatment arises from many different circumstances. Assessing these is an essential component of resolving the ethical dilemma. Ethically and legally, it is useful to distinguish between adults and young people. One of the characteristics of adulthood is personal responsibility for the way an adult chooses to live, even if this foreshortens life. In contrast, there is a widely accepted social responsibility to ensure that young people reach adulthood, at which point they take full responsibility for their decisions. Of course, the boundary between full adult responsibility and the ethical obligations to protect a young person is not marked by a single life event. There is a progressive capacity by young people to take responsibility for themselves. Any ethical analysis needs to take into account the gradual progression from an ethical obligation for adults to make decisions in the best interests of the child to increasingly showing respect for a young person's autonomy.

Jane is eight months pregnant and has been told that she has pre-eclampsia by her GP and should be admitted to hospital urgently for a Caesarean birth and treatment in order to protect her and the foetus from serious disability or death. Jane believes that serious illness and death are natural events that should not be interfered with. She refuses an emergency admission and instead asks to see the practice counsellor for personal support and insists on minimum medical intervention during the birth should she reach that point.

Here the doctor and counsellor share an ethical dilemma about their obligations to a pregnant woman and the foetus, which at this point has a reasonable chance of being a healthy baby after birth. If Jane is not mentally ill or being pressurized into this decision by others, then she is in the same position as any other adult with regard to accepting or refusing medical treatment. The doctor's ethical responsibility is substantially discharged by giving the patient adequate information to make an informed decision for herself (the requirements of the Mental Capacity Act 2005 and related Scottish law are considered later in this section). The counsellor's ethical position is no different from providing a service to someone who refuses medical intervention for any other illness. Respect for client autonomy is the ethical norm. However, this need not prevent the counsellor from exploring or even challenging the basis of the client's decision. Standards of practice consistent with the ethic of autonomy require that communicating alternative options takes place within a framework of respecting the client's right to make a decision for herself. It may also be appropriate to offer support in living with the consequences of that decision, as with any other client making a difficult and demanding decision.

The question of an ethical obligation to the potentially healthy baby within the mother is a separate issue but one that cannot be considered separately from the mother. Any ethical obligation to ensure the best interests of the foetus can be achieved only at the expense of violating the mother's autonomy and compelling her to undergo major surgery. This is an ethically contentious decision. There are credible arguments in favour of preserving the life of a viable foetus over a temporary violation of the rights of the mother. An alternative view is that the mother's autonomy is the ethical priority and takes precedence over the unborn child. There is no easy way of choosing between these alternatives. Either decision favours one at the significant expense of the other and raises questions about who carries the primary moral responsibility for making that decision. Courts have considered these circumstances. In some jurisdictions in the USA and Europe, the law prioritizes the preservation of life. In deciding in favour of the preservation of a baby's life, one judge explained that 'Where the harm is so great and the temporary remedy is so slight, the law is compelled to act ... Someone must speak for those who cannot speak for themselves' (*Winnipeg Child and Family Services v G*, 1997). The English legal tradition has taken different views on this issue.

There has been a case which showed how the court was prepared to intervene to save life if the judge could justify it. In *Re T* (Adult: refusal of treatment) [1993] 1 Fam 95, a judge made a declaration of lawfulness for a blood transfusion and a caesarean operation on a woman who was 34 weeks pregnant. She had been admitted to hospital following a road traffic accident. The Court of Appeal justified and rationalized the judge's order on the basis that, although the mother was an adult of sound mind and had refused the blood transfusion for religious reasons, on this occasion she was unable to make a rational decision at that time because she had been given the narcotic drug pethidine, her mother may have exerted pressure on her, and she had received some misleading responses to her enquiries about alternative treatments.

The Court of Appeal ([1992] 4 All ER 649 at 653) said in their judgment that although an adult patient was entitled to refuse consent to treatment irrespective of the wisdom of his decision, for such a refusal to be effective his doctors had to be satisfied that at the time of his refusal his capacity to decide had not been diminished by illness or medication or by false assumptions or misinformation, that his will had not been overborne by another's influence and that his decision had been directed to the situation in which it had become relevant; that where a patient's refusal was not effective the doctors were free to treat him in accordance with their clinical judgment of his best interests.

In a subsequent English case (*St George's NHS Trust v S*, 1998 at 692), the court affirmed other decisions that the mother's rights take precedence:

> In our judgement while pregnancy increases the personal responsibilities of a woman, it does not diminish her entitlement to decide whether or not to undergo medical treatment. Although human, and protected by law in a number of different ways … an unborn child is not a separate person from its mother. Its need for medical assistance does not prevail over her rights. She is entitled not to be forced to submit to invasion of her body against her will, whether her own life or that of the unborn baby depends on it. Her right is not reduced or diminished merely because her decision to exercise it may appear morally repugnant.

This case was of particular significance to counsellors and other caring professions because it also considered whether two doctors and a social worker had been correct in imposing a compulsory assessment order under mental health legislation and using that as the basis for seeking legal authority from a High Court judge to impose medical treatment. In the process of reaching a decision about these aspects of the case, the Court of Appeal concluded that the professionals had been wrong in law on two counts. First, the Mental Health Act cannot be used to achieve 'the detention of an individual against her will merely because her thinking process is unusual, even apparently bizarre and irrational, and contrary to the views of the overwhelming majority of the community at large.' Unusually in a law report, it is possible to gain some direct insight into the personal thinking of the woman who refused treatment as she recorded her objections to receiving treatment in writing. After giving her profession as veterinary nurse, and affirming her understanding of the medical consequences of the decision, she wrote:

> I have always held strong views with regard to medical and surgical treatments for myself, and particularly wish to allow nature to 'take its course' without intervention. I fully understand that, in certain circumstances, this may endanger my life. I see death as a natural and inevitable end point to certain conditions, and that natural events should not be interfered with. It is not a belief attached to the fact of my being pregnant, but would apply equally to any condition arising.

Second, a woman detained under the Mental Health Act cannot be forced into medical procedures unconnected with her mental condition unless her capacity to consent to such treatment is diminished. For example, a man suffering from schizophrenia has been legally supported in his decision to refuse to have a gangrenous leg amputated in the face of a medical consensus that it would be in his best interests and life-saving.

The importance of making a record of the basis on which it is decided that someone has the capacity to give or refuse consent to a proposed course of action also emerged in this case. The judgment criticized the doctors for failing to attend to their patient's capacity to consent or refuse consent to treatment. They concluded that 'None of the contemporary documents suggest that this factor was given express attention during the decision-making process.'

One of the aims of the Mental Capacity Act 2005 in England and Wales and the earlier Adults with Incapacity Act 2000 in Scotland was to clarify the law and to ensure compatibility with human rights law. This legislation sets out some core principles. A person over the age of 16 must be assumed to have the capacity to give valid consent until it is proved otherwise. This includes the right to refuse treatment for all persons over 18 years old and some rights to refuse for people aged 16–18. Someone must be supported to make a personal decision, as far as it is practicable to do so. Someone is not to be treated as lacking capacity simply because of making an unwise decision. Nor is capacity to be regarded as fixed or determined by a particular physical or mental characteristic or general ability to make decisions. Each assessment of someone's capacity must be made in the context of the decision to be made and may vary between different decisions.

Any relevant information to assist the making of a decision must be presented in ways that are appropriate to that person's circumstances. The assessment of whether someone has capacity depends on whether they can retain the information for long enough to make a decision and whether they are able to weigh it in order to arrive at a choice. Finally, someone must be able to communicate a choice even if it is restricted to blinking an eye to communicate 'yes' or 'no'. This development in law demonstrates a strong respect for individual autonomy and a robust protection of that right even when someone is in difficult circumstances due to illness or other limitations of their mental capacity. Further information can be found in Mitchels and Bond (2021), where capacity is considered in the context of client confidentiality and record-keeping, and consent is a fundamental issue. Updates and guidelines from government and charities can be found on the web.

The issue of a young person's right to refuse treatment is complicated by the progressive shift from total dependence on adults to self-reliance as adulthood approaches. Where the young person is considered incapable of giving or withholding consent, the responsibility for that decision rests with whoever holds parental responsibility. Where parental consent is being exercised against the young person's best interests or is unobtainable, the High Court may decide the appropriate course of action. Section 8 of the Family Law Reform Act 1969 gives 16–18-year-olds the right to consent to or refuse medical investigations and treatments. The courts have generally upheld these rights but have sought reasons to override the right to refuse treatment for life-threatening conditions. In *Re W* (1992) the Court of Appeal was considering the refusal of a 16-year-old suffering from anorexia to be transferred from one unit to another for treatment. The court decided that they could order her immediate transfer because they considered that anorexia had distorted the young person's ability to comprehend sufficiently to be able to rebut the rights given to her under the Family Law Reform Act. A similar decision was made in *Re J* (1992) where the issue of the power of a young person's ability to override parental consent was considered. In this case J was suffering from anorexia nervosa of such severity that there was a serious risk of irreversible damage to her brain and reproductive organs and her life was in danger. The Court of Appeal granted an emergency order enabling J to be treated despite her lack of consent. Although J maintained her refusal to consent, she accepted that the court order would have to be complied with. The Court of Appeal explained the decision in the following terms:

> No minor of whatever age has the power by refusing consent to treatment to override a consent to treatment by someone who has parental responsibility for the minor. Nevertheless such a refusal was a very important consideration in making clinical judgements and for parents and the court in deciding whether … to give consent. Its importance increased with the age and maturity of the minor. (Guardian Law Reports, 1992)

This view is consistent with an increasing emphasis in the law that the young person should be consulted and their views taken into account on any major decision about their best interests, even if they are deemed incapable of giving or refusing consent in their own right.

Below the age of 16, the ability to refuse investigations or treatment depends on an assessment of whether the child is of sufficient 'understanding and intelligence' (i.e. Gillick competent) to give or refuse valid consent. A fuller discussion of the assessment process can be found in Chapter 10 in relation to confidentiality. In the situation where a 'Gillick competent' young person gives consent, that consent cannot be vetoed by someone with parental responsibility. Conversely, a young person who is not considered to be 'Gillick competent' cannot veto valid parental consent. The counsellor or anyone else who provides a service or treatment on this basis is protected from legal action that might be brought on the grounds of invalid consent. The Master of the Rolls reiterated the protection given by a valid consent in the face of other objections to the proposed course of action (*Re W*, 1992 at 767). The valid consent may be withdrawn and this protection would cease unless other valid consents applied.

The legal framework creates a series of principles which have resulted in increasing recognition of the ethical value of respecting a young person's autonomy while balancing that with a general responsibility to act in the best interests of that young person. A theme which runs throughout the courts' decisions is reluctance to impose hard-and-fast rules that might be inappropriate to some cases. The decisions about the 'best interests of the young person' are made by considering all the relevant circumstances. Similarly, where an assessment of a young person's 'competence to give valid consent or refusal to consent' is required, that assessment would take into account the gravity of the decision to be made. In contrast, adults' right to refuse treatment is largely resolved by an ethic of respect for individual autonomy.

After a Death

It is increasingly common practice for counsellors to be called to give evidence in coroners' courts, especially about deaths where there is the possibility of suicide. The main aim of a coroner's court is to establish the identity of the deceased and determine the cause of death. If a counsellor is summoned to appear, it will usually be in order to establish the cause of death. This means that the counsellor will need to decide how much they are willing to say in open court. The central issue will be the agreement about confidentiality made with the client. It is accepted practice among counsellors that agreements about confidentiality should continue beyond a client's death.

It is often easier to discuss the nature of ethical difficulties outside a public hearing. For example, a counsellor might feel willing to answer questions in general terms about a client being depressed because of relationship difficulties, but may know there are some things which the client had stressed as being confidential, such as specific feelings about a named sexual partner or a relative. Most coroners will use their discretion in order to respect the ethical integrity of a professional witness where this does not compromise the purpose of the hearing. The coroner, who is usually a local doctor or solicitor, has considerable discretion about how they conduct the hearings. If any difficulties cannot be resolved by a preliminary discussion, it is advisable to seek legal advice and be legally represented in court.

After a suicide it is not unusual for relatives to want to discover whether everything had been done that could be done by those caring for the person who committed suicide. If they were unaware of the mental and emotional state of the person who died, they may also want as much information as possible. Out of their anger and grief they may wish to show that the counsellor was either incompetent or uncaring. This can lead to some challenging questions, either in court or elsewhere. It goes without saying that a counsellor who has been clear from the outset with a client about their qualifications, experience and policy over respect and autonomy or intervention to prevent suicide is in as strong a position as it is possible to be in these circumstances, particularly if they have also conducted an appropriate assessment in consultation with others and then acted on it. Evidence of clear agreement that either the client would abstain from suicidal attempts for the duration of counselling or that they would contact specified people or organizations should they become suicidal helps to add to the credibility of the counsellor and to an understanding of that counsellor's position with regard to client autonomy. Members of the general public, and particularly distressed relatives, may wrongly assume that a counsellor has a clear duty to intervene in all circumstances to prevent suicide, and may also have unrealistic expectations of what could have been done even if the counsellor did attempt to intervene.

The issue of keeping written **records** is highly relevant to any situation which might result in a court appearance. This is discussed in Chapter 15.

Conclusion

In this chapter, extensive reference to the law has been made. It is in the courts that the practical issues around the responsibilities of professionals towards people who are suicidal or are refusing life-saving treatment have been extensively examined. The courts have, in effect, become the venue for deciding public morality on these most contentious of cases. Different national jurisdictions have varied in the priority given to the ethical principles of respect for client autonomy or the preservation of life. Just as there is no universal agreement about which ethical principle should prevail in law, there are comparable divisions of opinion between counsellors about how best to respond. For some counsellors, the laws will reinforce their ethical convictions. Others will find the legal requirements contrary to their ethical convictions. Counsellors working in the UK need to take into account the legal framework that has been developed over many centuries since the assertion of personal liberty contained in Magna Carta. There is no general or automatic legal obligation to intervene on behalf of an adult who is suicidal or refusing medical treatment. Counsellors are working in a legal system that will usually support adults' rights to make decisions for themselves. The two most common circumstances likely to be encountered by counsellors where this is not the case concern adults who lack the capacity to give or withhold consent to psychiatric treatment due to a serious mental disorder under the provisions of mental health legislation or the complex provisions relating to young people and children. In the UK the law favours an ethic of respect for adult autonomy and protects an individual's right to consent to or refuse treatment as the usual basis for managing these difficult personal and social dilemmas.

The law that forbids actively assisting suicide, even in cases where someone is dying and wishes to avoid uncontrollable pain or a loss of control of their most basic bodily functions, is challenged in the media with increasing frequency, but there is little sign at the time of writing that assisting someone's autonomous choice to control the end of life can overcome concerns about the preservation of life or the risk of vulnerable people being pressurized into ending their lives.

This ethical analysis of how to respond to suicidal clients is organized around the principle of client autonomy, which helps to decide how to respond ethically and lawfully but cannot eliminate the unavoidable anxiety and anguish that are so often associated with death, especially for surviving relatives and social contacts.

Pause for Reflection

What do you consider to be the key ethical considerations for working with clients at risk of suicide in the context in which you practise? What steps have you taken to respond to these, and what discussions have you had with your supervisor about their expectations of you with respect to managing risk?

To access the online resources accompanying this chapter, please visit: https://study.sagepub.com/reevesandbond

8

Counsellor Competence

Chapter Overview

Competence is a basic ethical requirement for any counsellor. This chapter examines what is meant by competence and how it may vary between different therapeutic approaches, and particularly in the context of the scope of practice (SCoPEd consultation process). The legal distinction between competence and **negligence** is also considered. The chapter concludes by examining the relationship been competence and **impaired functioning** due to **illness** or **disability**.

Key words

competence, standard, **duty of care**, negligence, impaired functioning, disability, illness

A commitment by counsellors to work within their **competence** is widely recognized as fundamental to working ethically. It is one of the ethical requirements that not only recurs in the ethical **guidance** of national professional organizations (see Table 4.1) but also cascades down through **agency policy** and expectations that others hold of counsellors. Failing to work within one's own competence as a counsellor undermines many of the ethical principles considered essential to **counselling**. Clients are rendered vulnerable to additional emotional distress and psychological harm, the opposite of a commitment to doing good (**beneficence**) and avoiding doing harm (**non-maleficence**). The basis of **trust** between counsellor and client is undermined so that the counsellor becomes untrustworthy. Any claim to **respect** for client **autonomy** is discredited by the lack of basic respect being shown to the client's desire for enhanced self-determination. The counsellor is also working against their own interest by contradicting the ethical in ways that undermine **self-respect**. All of the six ethical principles that underpin counselling **ethics** are undermined by incompetence.

Therapist Competence

Professional competence requires having adequate skills, being properly qualified and trained as well as effective, and working ethically. The **responsibility** for ensuring competence rests on the individual counsellor in the last resort. No one else is better placed to monitor and evaluate whether counselling is being provided to adequate **standards**. It is not a purely personal self-assessment, but will be informed by feedback from clients, colleagues and professional **mentoring** or **supervision**. Some counsellors, especially those working in agencies, may use systematic audits of the client experience to inform awareness of issues of competence and where updating or training may be required. **Evidence-based** and **evidence-informed practice** is increasingly influential in determining what is considered best practice (see Chapter 16), but competence is still required even if the evidence for effectiveness is uncertain. Competence is a minimum standard for acceptable practice by the good-enough counsellor. Many will aspire to something above this level to achieve a standard between competence and excellence out of a sense of personal vocation or commitment and to obtain work in a competitive environment.

There are several complications in achieving competence: first, there is the process of becoming competent. A novice or trainee counsellor experiences the challenge of becoming competent most acutely, but how does someone know that they have reached this standard? Assessments by a trainer, service manager and/or supervisor are good guides here as well as self-monitoring. There is also that rather tricky transition to becoming competent between knowing enough to start seeing clients while still requiring support from someone who is more advanced in their development as a counsellor. The delivery of a competent level of counselling rests on a combination of individual ability and a systemic infrastructure of personal and professional development, so that responsibility for a competent service depends on several people, including the counsellor, until that counsellor is ready for more autonomous practice. This is not the end of the story when we have our competence as counsellors confirmed by qualifications, registration or accreditation. Every time we move into a new area of practice the cycle of learning begins again, from a state of 'not knowing' to competence.

Pause for Reflection

How do you know you are competent to work as a counsellor? What aspects do you draw on to inform your thinking and what mechanisms do you have in place to 'test out' your conclusions?

Sustaining competence requires a willingness to be self-critical and an awareness of changes to knowledge and practice in the field of counselling. The quest for competence is not a once in a lifetime achievement but recurs throughout the lifetime of counselling. It has to be assessed against a changing background of clients' needs and expectations in response to changes in society. Changes in the context of our work and the experiences we collect along the way, together with our own personal changes over our lifespan, mean we often have to relearn how to respond to familiar issues from new positions.

New technologies have opened up possible ways of delivering counselling that were inconceivable just a few years ago. Not only is the context within which counselling takes place changing, but so are the professional knowledge base and infrastructure to support competent practice. There is a perpetual need for updating, especially in the knowledge and skills base for practice, and increasingly to meet the demands of professional **accountability**.

Social Justice in Context

Through social movements, such as #metoo and #BlackLivesMatter, we are constantly challenged to reflect on ourselves, our context, viewpoints and perspectives that need to be reconfigured in the changing context of society. What was once viewed acceptable practice might no longer be viewed that way. Consider what active strategies you take to ensure that you remain open to challenge and change?

Scope of Practice

After three large professional associations entered into a formal collaborative process around 2016 (BACP, UKCP and BPC: for this section referred to as the Collaboration of Counselling and Psychotherapy Professions – CCPP), they quickly turned their attention to anomalies and problems in the field. These were multi-fold according to the CCPP and were negative undercurrents that prevented further progress in the development of professional practice. These included, in the context of the counselling professions not being statutorily regulated, difficulties in securing paid work for members, nor being able to implement national pay scales for counsellors; continuing debates around the similarities and differences between the terms 'counselling' and 'psychotherapy'; huge differences in training standards, from university-based Master's programmes through to two-day £19.99 programmes that claimed qualification, amongst others. The CCPP undertook a major scope of practice and education standards and, in that context, BACP stepped away from its long-held view of no difference between the terms 'counselling' and 'psychotherapy'; according to CCPP, the evidence pointed to there being a difference.

This scope of practice exercise, known by the abbreviation SCoPEd, went to all members of the CCPP (~70,000 practitioners) and in excess of 500 other stakeholder organizations in January 2019 – one of the largest consultation exercises undertaken by these Associations. While many were supportive of the key principles of the initial SCoPEd document, there were many opponents too, who argued SCoPED was: a power grab by greedy and inept professional organizations; introducing a false hierarchy into professional titles and thus undermining the integrity of many members; and was too aligned to a 'medical' model of 'illness', contrary to the underpinning philosophies of counselling.

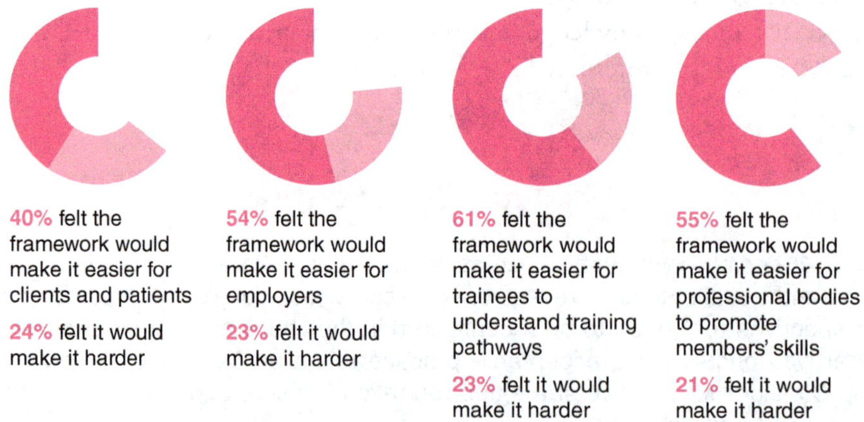

FIGURE 8.1 *Feedback summary from the first SCoPEd consultation*

At the time of writing, version 2 of the SCoPEd document was published, which is currently undergoing a second round of consultation. The titles of Counsellor, Advanced Counsellor and Psychotherapist were dropped, while critics claimed the core problems of the first document remained. Feedback for the first version of SCoPEd is summarized in Figure 8.1. There is no doubt that tackling some of the central problems of the profession were always going to be contentious and it remains to be seen whether SCoPEd in its current format will ultimately provide an answer to the problems identified by CCPP.

The mapping of evidence for SCoPEd covered several primary areas:

- Minimum teaching hours (direct tutor contact time).
- Minimum client or patient hours.
- Minimum supervision hours.
- Academic level of the qualification.
- Type of placement.
- Personal therapy requirements.
- Any additional requirements (e.g., BACP Certificate of Proficiency). (SCoPEd, 2020b: 10)

In summary, the SCoPEd framework identified clear differences in the 'points of entry' for the profession – the training and level of qualification that someone

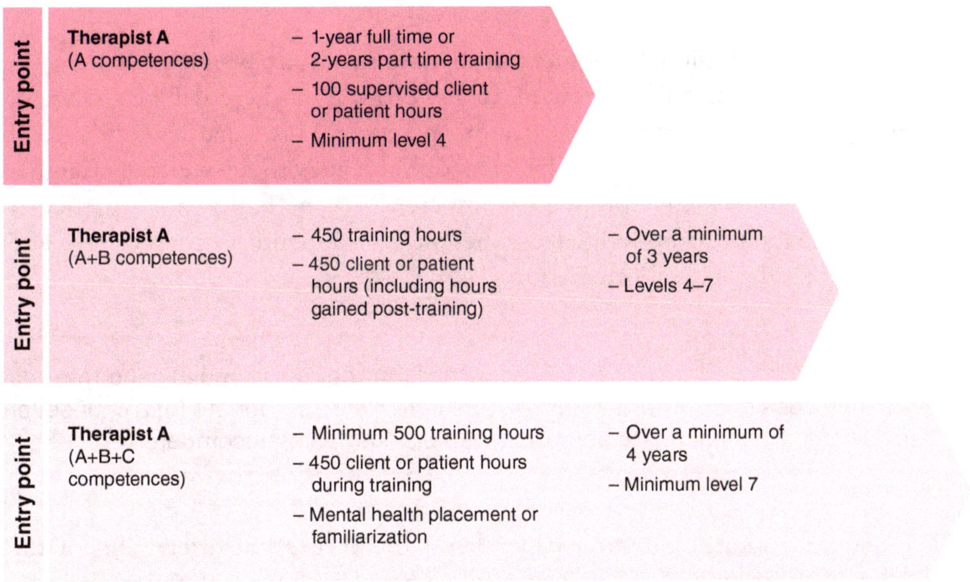

FIGURE 8.2 *A summary of competencies, training and practice requirements*

would undertake to become a qualified practitioner, but differences in practice were less clear. Competencies were identified across three primary areas, A, B and C – C being the 'highest' level. Figure 8.2 illustrates how training competencies were differentiated across the three areas.

The framework itself is too extensive to reproduce here, but can be found online via the BACP, UKCP and BPC websites. The consultation process, taking place at the time of writing, will take further time to evaluation before a third iteration is released. However, there is no doubt that SCoPEd might represent a sea-change in the counselling professions – for good or bad, depending on perspective – in terms of training standards and the competencies required to practise using a particular title, although, and certainly for the time being, there is no expectation of the counselling professions becoming statutorily regulated in the UK.

Pause for Reflection

What differences, if any, do you see in the work of counsellors and psychotherapists, and how best might clarity be achieved for clients accessing the services of those in the counselling professions?

Was My Counsellor Competent?

Concerns about professional judgment or incompetence are problematic for both clients and the professionals concerned. In any profession, there will be a range of opinions about what constitutes satisfactory practice. This is particularly true of counselling and can be illustrated by how difficult it is to answer the straightforward question 'Was my counsellor competent?'. Whether or not a particular intervention is likely to be judged competent will depend on the context and the counsellor's theoretical orientation.

'Kate is distressed by her counsellor telling her that he feels antagonistic towards her when she does or says certain things. She asks 'Is it appropriate for a counsellor to disclose that he feels angry and frustrated or is he being incompetent?'

The answer to Kate's question depends on the theoretical orientation of the counsellor. A different position will be reached based on how each theoretical orientation positions practice. Consider the four examples below.

From a *psychodynamic* perspective, such an intervention would be judged counterproductive. In order to help a client gain insight into their transferences, a counsellor deliberately keeps themself, as a human being, in the background. Jacobs (2010: 144) states that transference is partially resolved because:

> the counselling setting provides a chance for strong feelings to be expressed [by the client] for as long as is necessary, until they cease to exert so much pressure on the client … It is frequently the fear that love or hate drives others away that leads people to push down their strongest emotions. As they realize in counselling that the counsellor is not shocked, is not hurt, is not put off, does not misuse the client's feelings, or does not respond in any other inappropriate or damaging way – in other words, does not repeat the reaction which the client has experienced in the past – the very strength of the feelings can diminish.

The counsellor's interaction is therefore an act of incompetence in psychodynamic counselling.

However, this is not the view of a *person-centred* counsellor, whose objectives and methods are rather different. The person-centred counsellor focuses attention on the quality of the relationship between counsellor and client. Congruence is an essential quality in this relationship. Mearns et al. (2013: 13) say of congruence that 'The more the counsellor is able to be herself in the relationship without putting up a professional front or personal façade the greater will be the chance of the client changing and developing in a positive and constructive manner.' Therefore, the intervention could be highly appropriate and competent provided the counsellor's feelings are genuine and spontaneous, and communicated appropriately.

In *rational emotive* counselling this kind of **disclosure** would be more likely to be viewed as irrelevant. The type of self-disclosure recommended by Dryden and Neenan (2004: 19) is directed towards encouraging clients to internalize a new rational philosophy. The counsellor 'is to disclose not only how you as a counsellor have experienced a similar problem in the past, but also how you overcame it. Thus, for example, I sometimes tell my clients how I overcame my anxiety about having a stammer and therefore stammered less.' The counsellor's self-disclosure to Kate is not of this kind and is therefore irrelevant in rational emotive counselling. This sort of intervention would act as a distraction in *cognitive behavioural* counselling where the primary focus would be the client's cognitive processes (Trower et al., 2011). To the extent that the intervention disrupted the rapport between Kate and her counsellor, it could be judged more severely as both counterproductive and incompetent.

Not all counsellors are purists in the sense of adhering to a single model. Some, like Culley and Bond (2011), will seek to integrate skills drawn from a variety of models in a systematic way. From this viewpoint, a counsellor would be acting competently provided they were acting within the specific guidelines for the use of immediacy. If, on the other hand, the counsellor was randomly eclectic, there might well be no criteria for determining whether the intervention was competently executed.

A counsellor's theoretical orientation is only one of the contextual variations which might be relevant to assessing the competence of a particular intervention or method of working. The cultural setting, the needs of particular client groups, whether the counselling is one to one, with couples or in groups may also be relevant. What is competent in one context may be incompetent in another. This makes it difficult to generalize and to be specific and precise at the same time. Guidelines intended to have a wide application are of necessity written in general terms. For example, a general guideline that 'Counsellors should only disclose their immediate feelings about their clients when it is appropriate' might alert counsellors to a potential issue, but because it is written in terms that are intended for universal application it gives little actual guidance. It is easier to become much more specific once the context and particularly the theoretical orientation of the counsellor are established.

The Law and Competence

Any profession can learn from the experience of those courts that have long experience of hearing **negligence** claims that someone has provided seriously unsatisfactory service. 'Competence' is not a term that is much used in **law**. Lawyers have approached the issue of identifying adequate **standards** of practice from a different point of view. It is defined in terms of the service provider, including counsellors, having a duty to exercise 'due care', 'reasonable care' and/or 'reasonable skill'. It has been important in deciding claims for negligence to determine whether 'reasonable skill and care' have been used. Many of the leading cases relate to medical negligence where the courts have been faced with differences of view about what would constitute reasonable skill and care. Counsellors are not unique in having several established but conflicting views about how best to work.

What are *reasonable* skill and care? The same standards are not expected of a passer-by who renders emergency first aid after an accident compared to the skill of a qualified surgeon. Someone who is acting in a **voluntary** capacity may not be expected to show the same level of skill as someone who is working for reward. If someone practises a profession or holds themself out as having a professional skill, the law expects that person to show the amount of competence associated with the proper discharge of that profession, trade or calling. If that individual falls short of that standard and injures someone as a consequence, they are not behaving reasonably (Rogers, 2010).

How does a court assess what is a reasonable standard? The court will look to see if the counsellor explicitly promised a result as a term of the **contract** with the client. This is one of the reasons why counsellors are wise not to make such promises (e.g. to alleviate depression, anorexia etc., within a fixed time limit). In the absence of such a promise within a contract, the court will assess what constitutes a reasonable standard by using one of two procedures which will vary according to whether the court is dealing with professional or industrial procedures. It seems most likely that it is the professional procedure that would be used in cases relating to counselling.

If, as in counselling, there is no agreement about a universal standard of what is proper, then the court will not get involved in choosing between differences of professional opinion. The test is this: did the counsellor act in accordance with a practice accepted at the time as proper by a responsible body of professional opinion skilled in the particular form of treatment? It does not have to be a majority opinion in order to be valid. It is sufficient if the practices have been adopted by a minority of practitioners as demonstrating a reasonable level of care. Two other legal points may be particularly relevant to counselling.

First, the standard of reasonable skill and care requires striking a balance between the magnitude of the risk and the burden placed on the counsellor to avoid that risk. This may mean that a higher standard of care is required when the counsellor is working with issues about significant mental **illness**, HIV infection or abortion (or a high risk of potential **suicide**) compared to assertiveness or bereavement.

Second, there is a legal preference for associating a standard of care and skill with the post rather than with the individual who occupies it. In other words, courts expect the same minimum standard of a newly qualified counsellor as they would of an experienced practitioner in the same post. Similarly, no allowance is made for domestic circumstances or financial worries, or other factors which might contribute to error. This means that organizations are well advised to set the same standards for similar posts throughout their organization. For counselling in general, it is becoming increasingly important to establish a series of nationally recognized standards appropriate to different kinds of counselling posts.

In actual practice the courts are much less likely to become involved in hearing claims of negligence against counsellors than against services involving physical interventions, such as medicine, for the reasons outlined in Chapter 5. The difficulty that clients have in pursuing concerns about incompetent practice by counsellors through the courts and professional organizations places a considerable ethical responsibility on counsellors individually to assess whether they are working within their competence. The method of analysis used in law can help to inform the self-analysis process, but is insufficient by itself without the support of other strategies.

Enhancing Self-assessed Competence

One of the challenges faced by counsellors in determining adequate subjective standards of competence is the **privacy** of their work. Although the requirement of privacy is a widely held norm for counselling, it leaves the counsellor vulnerable to becoming isolated from the practice and the ideas of other counsellors in a way that is unlikely to happen in team settings where people work together. Therefore, it is desirable to develop strategies which will help to counteract a counsellor's isolation in standard-setting and to encourage that counsellor to inform their self-assessment by making reference to other counsellors.

The distinctive strategy that characterizes most of the reputable counselling movement is an emphasis on receiving regular and ongoing counselling supervision. This way of working together is distinguished from managerial supervision in order to create a relationship where the counsellor can talk frankly about issues of competence, personal doubts and vulnerabilities. As counselling supervision is such a distinctive ethical feature of counselling in the UK, it is discussed at greater length in Chapter 14.

Additional information about acceptable practice can be obtained from discussions with counsellors working in similar settings or with similar client issues. Membership of counsellor networks and associations takes on an ethical significance for counsellors who are working in isolation as a way of keeping in touch with acceptable practice. All the major professional organizations emphasize the importance of continuing professional development, which is usually achieved by periodically attending training conferences and courses. Further sources of information about what is currently considered to be competent practice are journals, books and, increasingly, the internet.

Counsellors with Impaired Functioning

One potentially very difficult situation has arisen from time to time and is, therefore, worth considering specifically. Like anyone else, counsellors are vulnerable to all the frailties of the human condition and these may affect their competence. Therefore, it is good practice that counsellors should not counsel when their function is impaired due to personal or emotional difficulties, illness, disability, alcohol, drugs, or for any other reason. It is reasonable to assume that most counsellors will know whether they have been drinking alcohol or taking drugs, medicinal or otherwise, which will then impair their functioning. Occasionally counsellors will be unaware of the effect of this consumption, particularly if they are becoming addicted.

There is another situation in which a counsellor's functioning may become impaired: the insidious erosion of ability due to illness or disability.

Trevor has a progressive illness that affects his conceptual abilities and he appears unaware that his interventions are increasingly confusing for clients. What is the responsibility of his counselling supervisor?

It is widely accepted that the counselling supervisor has a responsibility to raise the concern with Trevor and perhaps advise him to withdraw from counselling. Fortunately, this is a rare occurrence but there is a much more frequent variation of this situation which is less clear-cut.

Margaret has recently been bereaved by the death of her last surviving parent. She knows she is preoccupied with her loss. Should she withdraw from offering counselling?

This is the sort of situation that ought to be discussed in counselling supervision. Usually the counsellor will initiate the discussion, but the supervisor may take the initiative if the counsellor appears to be overlooking an important issue. There are four possible assessments of the situation:

1. The counsellor is able to use her current experience of bereavement as a resource for her clients, particularly those also experiencing bereavement.
2. The counsellor finds it too emotionally painful to function with recently bereaved clients but is able to continue working with other clients on non-bereavement issues.
3. The counsellor needs to withdraw temporarily from all counselling.
4. The counsellor needs to withdraw from providing counselling indefinitely or permanently.

Sometimes counsellors in situations such as those of Trevor or Margaret will be more optimistic about their ability to function than their counselling supervisor. Where there is a substantial difference of opinion and the counselling supervisor believes it is necessary to take positive action in the interests of protecting clients, the following procedure has proved useful:

1. The counsellor is told by their counselling supervisor of any reservations about their competence to practise, in writing if necessary.
2. If the counsellor and counselling supervisor cannot agree about the counsellor's competence, the opinion of a mutually acceptable third person is sought to make an assessment.
3. If the situation remains unresolved, the counselling supervisor may withdraw from that role, giving their reasons for doing so, which would usually be in writing.
4. The counselling supervisor may seek guidance from the counsellor's professional register or association or, in the last resort, implement the complaints or 'fitness to practise' procedure.

There is no suggestion that an individual should stop working as a counsellor because they have suffered a bereavement or have been ill or have developed an impairment such as hearing loss; fitness to practise depends entirely on a counsellor's ability to function effectively as a counsellor.

Conclusion

This brief review of ethical and legal significance indicates the advantages to counsellors and clients alike where counsellors can agree national standards for specific voluntary and professional posts. Guidance from professional bodies, latest **research** and current textbooks are all relevant sources for determining what is a reasonable level of practice.

There will always be a need for counsellors to monitor their own level of competence and be willing to be accountable to clients and other counsellors for their practice on a day-by-day basis. What can a counsellor do in these circumstances? Probably the minimum standard every counsellor should aspire to is made up of the following:

1. Know why you are doing or saying something to your client.
2. Be sure you are saying or doing what you intend.
3. Know what its effect is likely to be.
4. Adjust your interventions according to the client's actual response.
5. Review your counselling practice regularly in counselling supervision.
6. Develop strategies for keeping up to date and seek continuing professional development opportunities.

7. Assess whether your level of skill is the same or better than that of other counsellors offering counselling on similar terms or holding similar posts.

Simple as these principles are, they can act as the foundation for competent practice.

To access the online resources accompanying this chapter, please visit: https://study.sagepub.com/reevesandbond

9

Avoiding the Exploitation of Clients

Chapter Overview

This chapter considers the many different ways that clients are vulnerable to **exploitation**. It highlights examples of ideological, financial, sexual, emotional and professional pressures leading to client exploitation. It concludes by looking at essential safeguards in the form of powerful questions to challenge exploitation by ourselves as counsellors and by others.

Key words

exploitation, **respect**, ideological, financial, sexual, sexualized behaviour, emotional, professional

It is widely accepted that **exploitation** of clients is ethically incompatible with **counselling**. The use of the word 'exploit' carries with it strong negative moral overtones when applied to people, and especially when the exploitation takes place in a relationship founded on **trust**, **respect** for **autonomy**, and serving the best interests of the client. The difficult task is identifying the different forms of exploitation that can occur. The identification is much clearer when someone deliberately overrides their professional **values** and **ethics** but is less obvious when the exploitation is less premeditated or even wholly unintentional. The conventional classification of exploitation distinguishes between financial, sexual and emotional. To this list we could add ideological exploitation, such as the imposition of interpretations on a client's experience in order to validate the counsellor's belief system, whether that be political, economic, faith-based or philosophical, therapeutic position or otherwise.

Ideological Exploitation

It is unrealistic to expect a counsellor to perform the impossible task of suspending all personal beliefs in the interests of respecting client autonomy over their own beliefs (Adams, 2013). Any belief system pervades our experience of other people and ourselves, as well as influencing the way that we construct communications about these experiences. Some aspects of our belief systems must be present as an unseen influence between counsellor and client. Our beliefs and assumptions are in part shaped by our cultural and social backgrounds and our life stories. There may well be influences the other way, from client to counsellor, but the primary ethical interest, with regard to exploitation, is from counsellor to client. This raises the question of how these beliefs should be managed within counselling. There is a strong ethical argument that making therapeutically significant beliefs explicit is more respectful to the client than leaving them ill-defined in the undergrowth of the relationship. The ethical benefits of making a counsellor's position explicit are enhanced if that counsellor acknowledges the possibility of a client holding different beliefs and demonstrates respect for those beliefs.

Clive is in the midst of a painful separation from his partner that has led him to doubt his previously strong religious convictions. As he had contacted his counsellor through a religious network, he appears to assume that the counsellor is committed to the beliefs that he is now questioning. This assumption seemed of marginal significance when working on the break-up of the relationship, but the counsellor senses that Clive's assumption about his counsellor's beliefs may be discouraging Clive from exploring what his new beliefs might be and their impact on what he might want in future relationships.

This client is clearly at a critical moment of personal transition when his own beliefs are fluid and not yet secure in their formulation. This points to a need for care in how the counsellor influences the client's development of his beliefs.

The counsellor needs to be wary of viewing the client's dilemma as a corroboration of her own beliefs. If she were a strong believer, it would be ethically inappropriate to link the client's emotional pain with his crisis of faith and suggest that renewing his commitment to his former beliefs would alleviate his pain. This would be disrespectful of client autonomy and could be ideologically exploitative if this interpretation grows out of the counsellor's needs for bolstering her own belief system.

Conversely, it would be inappropriate for a counsellor who had abandoned her previously strong faith to seek to influence the client in that direction. More appropriate responses will depend on the therapeutic orientation of the counsellor. A psychodynamic counsellor may concentrate on exploring the significance of this client's assumption and fantasies about the counsellor's beliefs without either corroborating or disavowing these projections. The aim would be to legitimize the client's ownership and **responsibility** for developing his beliefs with greater insight into his own personal process. Humanistic and cognitive behavioural counsellors would be similarly interested in exploring the client's assumptions but might well follow this up with some personal **disclosure** of the counsellor's beliefs in the spirit of defusing the influence of the unknown and emphasizing the client's responsibility for reaching his own conclusions. Any or all of these interventions are fundamentally respectful of the client's autonomy and trust in the counsellor. It is arguable that passively continuing with the influence of the client's assumptions left unexplored is a less seriously exploitative act than co-opting the client's experience to corroborate the counsellor's beliefs. But it is a minor exploitation nonetheless. An opportunity to build the client's confidence and personal resourcefulness would have been missed, which might raise doubts about the **competence** of the counsellor. Questions about competence and autonomy are often entangled in any consideration of whether exploitation has occurred.

The first example of possible ideological exploitation has been chosen deliberately to focus on beliefs that might well be considered extraneous to counselling as it is usually practised. It is easier to see the ethical issues in these circumstances than where the belief system is intrinsic to the therapeutic model or position adopted by the counsellor. The ethical challenge posed by the 'false memory' versus 'recovered memory' debate concerns the counsellor imposing a predetermined view that abuse has or has not taken place as a matter of personal belief or ideology in ways that pre-empt the client's own search for memories and their interpretation. The pre-empting tendency is so powerful in this instance that there is no widely accepted term for a client who discovers previously 'lost' memories of sexual abuse within counselling or therapy. As Jenkins (1996, 2012) pointed out in his informative analysis of the ethical and legal implications of the debate surrounding this issue, both 'false memory syndrome' and 'recovered memory' are terms with inbuilt persuasive tendencies towards partisan positions within the debate. The former seeks to exclude the possibility that any such memory could be based on actual instances of sexual abuse and usually attributes the phenomenon to the insidious influence of the counsellor or therapist who implanted the memory and its interpretation, leading to false accusations against family members. Conversely, the term 'recovered memory' suggests **acceptance** that the memory is invariably based on historical fact. In the absence of less loaded terms, perhaps the terms 'tentative' and 'corroborated' should be used to distinguish between memories that have an unknown historical basis and those that have been confirmed independently of the client.

Angela reveals during her counselling that she has some 'blank periods' in her memory of her childhood when she cannot recall where she was or what happened. She has a sense that something terrible happened and has heard from friends that this could be an indication of having been sexually abused. She realizes that these 'lost memories' coincide with her mother ending a relationship with her natural father and starting a relationship with her stepfather, with whom she has never had a close relationship. As a result of her concern about the significance over the 'blank periods', the relationship with her stepfather has worsened from merely being distant to open hostility, with negative effects on her relationship with her mother. She wants to resolve the issue of these missing memories.

In a situation like this, there is no corroboration of any sexual abuse. The client has some indications that may suggest some form of trauma that need not necessarily be the consequences of sexual abuse. Few counsellors can come to situations of this kind without being mindful of the controversy evoked in our own profession by Freud, changing his views from hysteria being founded on historical events of abuse to having its origins in fantasy (Masson, 1985; Mitchels, 2006: 76–9). Awareness of the early history of psychoanalysis and its societal and subsequent theoretical struggles with the possibility of sexual abuse indicates the level of difficulty that suspicions of sexual abuse pose for therapy. Personal experience is very powerful, perhaps the most powerful influence on the counsellor's predisposition towards seeking to corroborate or doubt the occurrence of sexual abuse. Counselling ethics do not stop a counsellor holding strong personal convictions about this or any other issue. However, the application of counselling ethics would point to the importance of keeping any personal convictions bracketed out of helping a client resolve lost memories. Memories can be fragile and overridden by inappropriate interventions. The challenge is supporting the client in exploring memories and preserving their integrity.

Issues around eating disorders can also present challenges. There has been a persistent view in the mental health field over the years that all eating disorders have their origins in sexual abuse and, more specifically, that all bulimia (i.e. gorging and vomiting food) is the result of oral sexual abuse. It is important to keep in mind that eating disorders may or may not be associated with sexual abuse. It seems equally important to avoid contaminating a client's material by imposing this interpretation in order to sustain a therapeutic ideology. It is ethically better to bear in mind the many different theoretical explanations of the origins of eating disorders and to be open-minded as to which one will most closely fit any particular client's experience.

Ideological exploitation is not only harmful to clients and others who may be implicated by invalidated accusations, but also discredits the validity of counselling and therapy. Whenever a therapeutic theory suggests a general belief that 'a is caused by b', there are ethical issues about the application of that theory in work with individual clients and the degree of respect shown to clients in determining whether that belief is confirmed or contradicted by their experience. For example, if the client is recalling actual sexual abuse, the respectful starting point is to believe what the client is saying rather than to doubt without good cause. Pathologizing solely on the basis of therapeutic theory or personal beliefs what has its roots in real events is arguably another form of ideological exploitation or abuse.

Social Justice in Context

Ideological exploitation could be described as a social justice issue. The often-encountered power imbalance between counsellor and client, as has been discussed elsewhere in this book, increases the potency of a counsellor's beliefs and how they might, inadvertently, be asserted over the client. If counsellors do not undertake careful reflection of their personal beliefs, or upbringing, surrounding race, culture, sexual identity, age and disability, for example, the very real danger of causing harm through positions taken in therapy can be profound.

Financial Exploitation

The potential for financial exploitation in counselling occurs in a number of ways. The most common source of complaint arises from a lack of clarity about the financial costs incurred by clients.

Stephanie seeks counselling and agrees to a fee of £30 per session. After the first two months she and the counsellor agree to meet more frequently and change from fortnightly sessions to weekly. The discussion about the new arrangements was hurried and at the end of a session. Some time later, Stephanie is perplexed and shocked to receive a bill for £160 at the end of the next month. She had wondered what the cost would be, but had calculated that the maximum charge would be for four weekly meetings at £30, a total of £120. When she raised the issue, her counsellor explained that his charges had gone up to £40 per session at a point during the first two months of seeing her and, as this was a new arrangement, he felt obliged to charge at the higher rate.

This is a classic example of where a lack of clarity about fees, prior to the client incurring costs, can lead to a misunderstanding and even destroy trust in the counselling relationship. It would have been better if the original arrangement had been an agreed fee for a fixed amount of counselling expressed in hours or sessions. This would have removed uncertainty about the implications of any changes in arrangements. Any increase in charges without notice and charged retrospectively is arguably exploitative. It is also unenforceable in **law**. One of the basic requirements of a legally valid **contract** is prior agreement about its terms.

Clients are entitled to feel cheated if, after reaching an agreement about the payment, the counsellor is bad at time-keeping, particularly if this results in the client paying a full fee for a session when they have only received part of one. Habitually bad time-keeping is almost certainly an indication of low standards of practice by a counsellor. However, like anyone else, a counsellor can be unexpectedly delayed by an accident or for some other reason. This might also be the case in the event of technical issues encountered when delivering therapy online, for example the therapist's internet connection failing during the session. What should a counsellor do in these circumstances? The obvious course of action is to reduce the fee in proportion to the time missed. If, however, the purpose of the session has been frustrated by this shortage of time, then it may be more appropriate to make no charge. If a client has incurred costs or been inconvenienced to attend a session which has been adversely affected by the time-keeping of the counsellor or even their total absence, then it may be more appropriate to reimburse those costs and sometimes to pay compensation. One way of minimizing inconvenience to a client is to have a prior agreement about how long that client should wait for the counsellor before assuming the session is abandoned. Such an agreement would only apply when something unexpected has intervened. It is much better to avoid such situations and if a session needs to be rescheduled to have reached an agreement about the new arrangements as far as possible in advance.

Counsellors who charge fees for their services are vulnerable to the suspicion that they keep fee-paying clients on longer than is strictly necessary. There are two opposing views about who is responsible in this situation. Some take the view that it is the client's responsibility to monitor whether or not they want to continue counselling and whether they are getting value for money. This seems appropriate when the counselling is clearly provided on this basis and the counsellor does not express an opinion about the desirable duration of the counselling relationship. It is arguably another way of respecting client autonomy. However, in practice, matters are not always as clear-cut as this.

Polly values her counselling sessions, which started when she was having difficulties due to bereavement. She asks her counsellor how long she is likely to benefit from counselling. He replies that in his experience of comparable situations six months would be the appropriate length. In the event Polly makes more rapid progress and after two months has begun to use the sessions to consider other aspects of her life. She is fee-paying and always pays willingly, which is a relief to her counsellor, who is experiencing financial difficulties.

In these circumstances it is more appropriate for the counsellor to draw attention to a change in the purpose of the sessions and to reach a new agreement. The temptation is to allow the counselling relationship to extend itself by the counsellor's inaction to the end of six months or indefinitely. The tendency to extend contracts with wealthy clients is not always deliberate. One way counsellors can check whether this is actually happening is by monitoring whether they give wealthy clients longer contracts than their poorer clients, and by periodically reviewing this issue in counselling **supervision**. Incorporating periodic reviews with clients about their counselling contracts also acts as a safeguard. It is a test of the counsellor's integrity whether they can set aside their financial needs in order to negotiate the duration of the counselling relationship so as to take into account the client's best interests.

Sometimes clients will want to give their counsellor a gift. This raises issues that involve the integrity of both the counselling relationship and the counsellor.

Elsie is alienated from her relatives and wishes to leave her counsellor a substantial sum of money in her will.

This situation could threaten the integrity of the counselling relationship if the client's conscious or unconscious intention is to buy the counsellor's loyalty or manipulate the relationship in some way. On the other hand, it could be a straightforward way of acknowledging the personal value that the client places on the counselling, which will only take effect once the relationship is over. The risk to the counsellor's integrity is the suspicion that they may have used their influence to obtain the gift. For all these reasons, counsellors are wise to be cautious about accepting gifts and to refuse to do so if this would compromise the counselling relationship. If there are no obvious reasons for declining the gift, it is a sensible precaution to protect the counsellor's reputation to discuss it in counselling supervision, and in the case of a substantial gift, to discuss this with their professional association. Often it is more appropriate to encourage the client to make a gift to charity rather than to the counsellor personally.

Sometimes financial exploitation may arise from dual relationships operating concurrently between the counsellor and client.

Douglas, a car dealer, knows that his counsellor wants to buy a car. After some negotiation, the counsellor agrees to purchase a car from Douglas. In the event, the car turns out to be faulty and they are unable to agree on how to resolve it. She then sues Douglas.

This case reveals that there are many dangers in dual financial relationships. At the very least the counsellor has left herself vulnerable to the suspicion that she has used her role in relationship to Douglas to obtain a more favourable deal from Douglas than she could obtain elsewhere. Even if this were not the case, the potential for the business transaction undermining the counselling relationship is a high one if grievances arise in the commercial relationship. It is very unlikely that the dual relationships, counselling and financial, could be kept separate. In the example, it is the client's part of the deal that is problematic, but the effect would be much the same if the counsellor had difficulty making payments or if any of many other possibilities arose.

Sometimes counsellors will enter into dual relationships out of the best intentions.

Jon is a fee-paying client in the middle of his counselling when he is made redundant. His counsellor agrees to Jon's offer of doing odd jobs for him instead of paying fees.

There are dangers in this situation for both counsellor and client. What if the counsellor is dissatisfied with Jon's work? On the other hand, what is a reasonable rate of pay from Jon's point of view? The potential difficulties are such that both these situations need to be considered in advance of entering into such an arrangement. Some counsellors prefer to avoid the risk of such complications by using a sliding scale of fees that could be adjusted according to Jon's circumstances, or by continuing counselling without any charge.

Bartering goods is sometimes considered as an alternative arrangement in circumstances similar to Jon's. What if Jon agrees to give the counsellor an ornament or some other possession as an alternative method of payment? Again, the **problems** are similar to bartering services. The counsellor needs to consider in advance what would happen if the object exchanged turns out to be damaged or faulty. Jon needs to be confident that he is getting value in the exchange. Probably an independent valuation is required as the starting point for any agreement. It is unclear if there are any UK guidelines for situations where fees are paid by barter (although there might be professional ethical considerations around the existence of dual roles). In the USA, these issues have received more extensive attention (see Herlihy and Corey, 1992). The American Counseling Association makes the following provision about bartering in its *Code of Ethics*:

> Counselors may barter only if the relationship is not exploitive or harmful and does not place the counsellor in an unfair advantage, if the client requests it, and if such arrangements are an accepted practice among professionals in the community. Counselors consider the cultural implications of bartering and discuss relevant concerns with clients and document such agreements in a clear written contract. (ACA, 2014: A.10.e)

Sexual Exploitation

Social awareness of sexual exploitation and harassment by people with power over others has increased dramatically over the last decade. It is widely accepted that there is a significant amount of sexual abuse of children by adults, often members of their own family. There is also a growing realization that members of the caring professions, including psychiatrists, psychologists, social workers and counsellors, have also engaged in sexually inappropriate behaviour with their clients (Rutter, 1989; Russell, 1993, 1996; Jehu, 1994).

There are no means of knowing accurately how frequently clients suffer sexually inappropriate behaviour but there are indications that it is sufficiently frequent to be a real cause for concern. In the USA, it was estimated that sexual contact occurs between male therapists and clients in about 11% of cases and between female therapists and clients in 2–3% of cases (Pope and Bouhoutsos, 1986). A subsequent downturn in self-reported cases by therapists may indicate that increased awareness of the issue has been successful in reducing sexually inappropriate behaviour. On the other hand, it may be the result of less candid self-reporting (Pope and Vasquez, 1991).

In the UK, the incidence is less certain. They are a significant but minority source of complaints in BACP professional conduct procedures between 1996 and 2006 (Khele et al., 2008). It appears that incidents are under-reported. Even if the incidence of sexual misconduct by counsellors turns out to be lower than in the USA, and there is no evidence to suggest that this is the case, more needs to be done to reduce it further. The effect on clients is so devastating that their reactions have been likened to the victims of rape, battering, incest, child abuse and post-traumatic stress syndrome. Pope (1988) has described the therapist–patient sex syndrome as involving many of the features of these other traumas:

- *Ambivalence*: A state of fearing separation or alienation from the counsellor, yet longing to escape their power and influence. For as long as the ambivalence persists, the client may not report the counsellor out of a sense of loyalty and fear of destroying their professional reputation.
- *Guilt*: This arises because the client may feel responsible for not having stopped the sexual activity or for having initiated it. However, it is the counsellor's responsibility to monitor the **boundaries**, even if the client does act seductively, and it is the counsellor who is responsible for maintaining the appropriate level of personal/professional distance, not the client. The client's sense of guilt is often similar to the feelings associated with child abuse and there is a similar sense of responsibility for what happened on the part of the client.
- *Emotional lability*: A long-term consequence of counsellor–client sexual involvement can be a sense of being emotionally overwhelmed during the relationship, which may be followed by periods of emotional instability. Sometimes the emotional volatility occurs inappropriately with sexually appropriate partners.

Other responses identified by Pope include **identity**/boundary/role confusion, sexual confusion, impaired ability to trust, suppressed rage, cognitive dysfunction, and increased suicidal risk. The risk of serious emotional distress to the client is only one of the reasons why there appears to be universal prohibition on sex with clients by national professional bodies for counsellors. There are other reasons why sex between counsellors and clients is considered dangerous. Clients are vulnerable to exploitation because of the inequality of power that is inherent in a counselling relationship. Inevitably, the helper will hold more power than the person being helped will. It is the difference between being the provider and the needy. Psychodynamic counsellors have also pointed out the likelihood of a powerful transference growing between the client and counsellor arising from the client's childhood. When this occurs, the client is relating emotionally to the counsellor as a child would to an adult or a parent. If the counsellor enters into a sexual relationship, it is experienced as sexual abuse or incest. This may explain the level of distress experienced by some clients.

The risks inherent in sex with clients are not confined to the client's reaction. The public reputation of counselling in general is at stake. The public must have confidence that they can approach counsellors and discuss personal issues in a safe environment. As part of the counselling process people often become emotionally vulnerable and expose themselves psychologically to their counsellor. Therefore, it is important that the counsellor maintains an appropriate boundary in the relationship to provide the client with **safety**. The 'no sex' rule for counsellors is out of respect for the clients' psychological vulnerability in the same way as doctors need to respect their patients' physical vulnerability. The prohibition on sex with clients therefore both protects current clients and also protects the reputation of counselling in the public mind so that future clients feel able to take the risk of approaching a counsellor.

What are sexual activity and sexualized behaviour?

The prohibition of sexual activity with current clients was adopted in the first BAC *Code of Ethics and Practice for Counsellors* in 1984, and repeated in subsequent ethical guidance not only from BACP but also from COSCA, BPS, IACP and UKCP. This prohibition is applied internationally by counselling organizations and has inevitably raised the question 'What is sexual activity or a sexual relationship?' The phrases imply that the ethical concerns extend beyond sexual intercourse involving penetration to include other behaviours, such as masturbation, 'heavy petting' and so on. But where is the boundary between sexual activity and hugging and kissing, which are activities that may or may not have an obvious sexual component? The sexual ambiguity of these activities means that it is impossible to produce a clear definition of what constitutes sexual activity. With some activities, it will depend on the intention of the people involved and, just as importantly, the interpretation of the person on the receiving end. Counsellors are wise to be cautious in situations where their actions can be misunderstood.

Advice from the Council for Healthcare Regulatory Excellence (2008) on clear sexual boundaries uses the term 'sexualised behaviour' to include behaviours that have sexual overtones but are not necessarily thought of as sexual activities. Such behaviour is forbidden for all healthcare workers because of its potential to:

- cause significant and enduring harm;
- damage trust;
- impair professional judgment.

Examples of sexualized behaviour (adapted to be relevant to counselling) include:

- asking for or accepting a date;
- using sexual humour during consultations;
- making inappropriate sexual or demeaning comments or asking irrelevant questions, for example about a patient's/client's body, underwear, sexual performance or orientation;
- requesting details of sexual orientation, history or preferences that are unnecessary or irrelevant;
- asking for, or accepting an offer of, sex;
- the unnecessary exposure of the either the client's or counsellor's body during the consultation;
- hugging or touching that is inappropriate;
- having meetings outside counselling sessions with a sexual intent;
- keeping or taking photographs or other **records** of a client for the sexual pleasure of the counsellor;
- undertaking any act that is for the counsellor's sexual gratification (including grooming in preparation for such an act);
- exchanging drugs or services for sexual gratification;
- a sexual assault.

In terms of helping counsellors to think through the issues around sex with clients, it is useful to list these different activities separately and realize that any sexualized activity with a client is likely to fall into one of these categories.

'Sexual and sexualized activity' also has positive connotations associated with intimacy, physicality and relationships, and outside of the counselling relationship can be extremely positive and life-enhancing. The prohibition on sex between clients and counsellors is not based on latter-day puritanism but on the expectation that both counsellor and client should look to others for sexual fulfilment independent of each other. Counsellors who have entered into sexual relationships with clients could be argued to fall into several distinct categories. There are a few who deliberately use counselling as a means of obtaining sexual contacts and who appear relatively indifferent to what happens to the client afterwards. Their motivation and behaviour are pathological. More often, counsellors who cross the boundary do so because of a lack of satisfactory emotional and sexual relationships in their own lives. Such a person may well use clients (and trainees) as a source of social company and hence the possibility of sexual relationships is increased. Counsellors behaving in this way often have considerable confusion over issues to do with personal boundaries, which may permeate much of their life and their work with clients. The best way a counsellor can avoid this situation is to explore their own sexual needs and ensure that they satisfy these needs outside their counselling relationships. A counsellor who has done this is in a much better position to deal with the sexual attraction that will inevitably arise from time to time.

Sexual attraction

Sometimes it will be the client who feels the sexual attraction most strongly and who clearly takes the initiative in attempting to seduce the counsellor. Does this make the counsellor responding positively any less problematic or exploitative? The counsellor's role here is to acknowledge the sexual experience of the client, but to do so such that it facilitates the client's capacity for relationships outside of the therapeutic relationship. 'No' can be a therapeutic word.

Protecting the integrity of the counselling relationship

Jack appreciates the help he has received and has become attracted to his counsellor. How should his counsellor react when he invites him to meet outside the counselling sessions?

When a client appears to be sexually attracted to a counsellor, it is important to be clear about the purpose and boundaries in counselling. Rather than comply with the client's overtures, it is better to acknowledge openly what appears to be happening and then explore what the client wants from a sexual relationship with the counsellor. If this situation is handled well, it often marks the movement into a new phase in counselling where both the client and counsellor feel able to discuss their feelings about each other more directly. It is often a time when the client is willing and able to disclose personal needs more frankly, which are not being met elsewhere in their lives. For the counsellor, it is important that this kind of situation is discussed in counselling supervision so that they feel clear about, and supported in, maintaining an appropriate professional boundary. Any alternative approach is usually less satisfactory.

To pretend to ignore a client's advances represents avoidance of where the greatest energy in the relationship may be currently operating, and with it the greatest motivation to work on real needs and issues. To comply with the advances and become involved in sexual activity not only defuses and misdirects potential therapeutic energy, but also carries with it personal risks for both the counsellor and client. For the counsellor, in the event of a complaint, there is also the likelihood of their expulsion from professional associations.

If we experience pain or a sense of loss in declining the advances of a client, then that ought to be a prompt to discuss what is happening in supervision or a prompt for our own therapy. Sometimes the psychological intimacy of counselling can conceal a counsellor's own unmet needs. Keeping the focus on the integrity of the counselling relationship with the client can be challenging in many different ways and sometimes may cast a spotlight on the counsellor's needs and desires in unexpected and uncomfortable ways. Avoiding client exploitation requires meeting those needs outside the work with clients.

Counsellors can also sometimes experience a powerful sense of sexual attraction towards a client. It is still probably taboo to talk about such feelings (Pope et al., 2006). If we have not experienced such feelings, we can imagine the feelings we might experience if we encounter a client who is our sexual ideal and who also has personal qualities we admire. Sometimes extremely strong sexual attractions can develop in longer counselling relationships of a psychologically intimate nature. The desire to move into a sexual relationship may be enormous. It is not unethical to feel attraction to a client. The ethical response is to acknowledge the feeling to ourselves and to then consult a counselling supervisor and colleagues about the situation as quickly as possible. The decision about whether to tell a client about our feelings of attraction will be a matter of judgment depending on the circumstances and the model of counselling being used. Sometimes seeking our own counselling can prove useful. It is probably the case that comparatively few counselling training programmes include any formal training in how to recognize and respond to sexual attraction in counselling. This is a serious omission.

Sex with former clients

It is only comparatively recently that the issue of sexual relationships with former clients has started to receive serious consideration by counsellors on both sides of the Atlantic. Debate around this issue gained momentum during the mid-1990s, within the BACP (Bond, 1994) and BPS (Jehu, 1994). The BACP's current position is summarized in its *Ethical Framework* for counsellors:

> We will avoid sexual or intimate relationships with former clients or people close to them. Exceptionally, such a relationship will only be permissible following careful consideration in supervision and, whenever possible, following discussion with experienced colleagues or others concerned about the integrity of the counselling professions, when:
>
> - enough time has elapsed or the circumstances of the people concerned have sufficiently changed to establish a distinction between the former and proposed new relationship
> - any therapeutic dynamics from the former relationship have been sufficiently resolved to enable beginning a different type of relationship.

(This may not be possible with some clients or inappropriate to some therapeutic ways of working.)

- an equivalent service to the one provided by the practitioner is available to the former client, should this be wanted in future
- the practitioner has taken demonstrable care in ensuring that the new relationship has integrity and is not exploitative. (BACP, 2018a: 18)

One of the challenges in reaching an agreed policy was an issue that divides counsellors according to the nature of the work they do with clients and a counsellor's theoretical orientation. Some examples may illustrate these different widely held opinions.

Lesley seeks counselling to help her to manage a conflict between her and a colleague at work better. A combination of problem solving and assertiveness techniques is successful. After two counselling sessions she has resolved her problem and the counselling stops. Six months later she bumps into her counsellor socially at a party and after a pleasant evening together they decide to meet socially. Neither person is in a relationship with someone else. Some weeks later they start a sexual relationship.

In this example, the counselling work is unlikely to have involved much intimacy or intensity as the theoretical orientation has a strong behavioural component and the focus of the work is outside the immediate counsellor–client relationship. The meeting that precedes the sexual relationship also occurs in a setting unconnected with the counselling and on equal terms. It seems inappropriate to prohibit two adults from continuing to develop their relationship in the way they want in these circumstances. It has been argued that to be too protective of clients is to infantilize them and constitutes an erosion of their autonomy. Counsellors who believe this situation is typical argue against any restraint on sex with former clients or for minimal restraints.

David uses counselling to explore his difficulty in having close relationships that last longer than a few months. During the counselling, which was weekly over five months, attention is paid to his feelings towards his counsellor, Sam, who points out when he feels David is trying to distance himself from him. As a result, David becomes aware of how he pushes people away and how this re-enacts a painful period during his childhood. Six months after the end of the counselling David meets Sam at a charity event and suggests they meet again for a meal. Both of them realize that there is a mutual sexual attraction. What should Sam do?

In this example the counselling was more intense, intimate and longer-lasting. This is the kind of situation where powerful transferences and counter-transferences are likely to arise, whether or not the counsellor is using a psychodynamic model, and considerably greater caution is required before a sexual relationship is started, if ever. For example, members of the College of Sexual and Relationship Therapists (CORST) (2019) have adopted a ban on sexual relationships with former clients. They believe this is essential to protect the integrity of counselling on these sorts of issues. There is anecdotal evidence that some clients are deterred from seeking counselling about relationship and sexual issues because they are not confident that counsellors will not engage in sex with them. Many practitioners with a psychodynamic orientation also doubt whether it would ever be possible to enter into a relationship that is truly free of the transferences and power dynamics of the original counselling. This is the focus of one of the debates that is currently taking place. Should the prohibition on sex with former clients be absolute and forever? Alternatively, is it possible that in some situations, transferences are resolved and therefore it becomes a matter of judgment whether sex with a former client is permissible? The kinds of criteria to be taken into consideration are:

- Has sufficient time elapsed to mark a clear boundary between the counselling and the new relationship? (The American Counseling Association requires a minimum of five years: ACA, 2014: A5c.)
- Have the dynamics involved in the counselling, particularly with special attention to power and transference, been given careful consideration by the counsellor, and are there good reasons for believing these are resolved and no longer influential in the proposed relationship?
- Have the risks to the client been explored with them?
- Has the issue been discussed with the counselling supervisor and their support for the relationship been obtained?

If the counsellor decides to go ahead with starting a sexual relationship after satisfying these requirements, they need to be aware of the possibility of the former client experiencing many of the symptoms of the therapist–patient syndrome described earlier. Because of this, most prudent counsellors would prefer to avoid sex with former clients unless the counselling relationship had been extremely brief, lacking in emotional intensity, and therefore not involving the dynamics of transference and power which might persist or recur in a subsequent non-counselling relationship. Using these criteria, it would be personally and professionally prudent of Sam to avoid entering into a sexual relationship with David.

Pause for Reflection

Do you believe sexual relationships can be appropriate with clients if there has been minimal therapeutic engagement? What informs your thinking?

Counselling in an appropriate environment

Rowan (1988: 26) has drawn attention to the way the furnishings of a counselling room communicate to a client what is expected of them. He suggests, for example, that 'Cushions on the floor give much more flexibility and a suggestion that it is alright to be childlike or even childish. And a couch or mattress lends itself to fantasy, dreams, deep regression and loss of conscious rational control.' In contrast, it is argued that chairs suggest rationality and the straighter the chair, the greater the emphasis on rationality. Similarly, the presence of a box of tissues may be perceived as indicating that others have used the room for crying and that the counselling room is a safe place to cry in.

Without wishing to press these observations too far, probably most counsellors would recognize a degree of reality in these and acknowledge the conscious and unconscious influence of the physical environment in which counselling takes place. One of the obvious questions which follows is, why do some counsellors see clients in either the counsellor's or the client's bedroom? This must send mixed messages about a counsellor's intentions. It is better to avoid counselling in bedrooms altogether. If this is not possible, it is better to use a room that is not being used regularly by the counsellor or client, such as a spare room and optimally a dedicated room for counselling that is appropriately furnished for the type of counselling to be undertaken. An obvious exception to this is when counselling someone who is confined to bed because of illness.

Emotional Needs

Much of what has already been said about sexual exploitation is directly transferable to emotional needs. If the boundary in sexualized activity is sometimes hard to identify, this is even more so with emotional needs. This is not problematic if the need is complementary to the client's use of counselling and is sufficiently within the counsellor's control to avoid distorting the counselling relationship. A counsellor's emotional needs are not always counterproductive. Sometimes a counsellor's neediness or vulnerability can be used as a resource in order to enhance a client's understanding of their own situation or to break down a sense that the client is unique in experiencing a particular vulnerability. This often represents a high standard of practice and is within the tradition of the 'wounded healer'. The problem arises when the counsellor's neediness is such that the client's needs are eclipsed, or under the pretence of working to meet a client's needs, the counsellor is really seeking satisfaction of their own. This can occur in a huge variety of ways. The most obvious are counsellors who cannot end relationships with clients because they are a source of regular companionship and a substitute for the counsellor developing friendships with people who are not their clients. Perhaps a little less obvious is the counsellor who has such a sense of personal unworthiness that they choose to work with the most socially stigmatized and disadvantaged clients available to them on the basis that at least they will be grateful for help. Often, however, they will not be grateful or appreciative, and the counsellor's disappointment and sense of rejection can become the dominant emotional force in the relationship rather than the client's feelings of vulnerability.

Good practice with regard to emotional exploitation requires that counsellors periodically review what their emotional satisfactions and needs are. It is important that the counsellor has alternative sources of emotional satisfaction from outside counselling for most of their deep needs. Good quality counselling supervision is invaluable in helping counsellors address this issue.

Powerful Questions against Exploitation

There are number of powerful questions we can ask ourselves to expose exploitation in the work we are undertaking:

- Whose interests are being served?
- Who benefits most from this approach to counselling?
- When the counselling is completed whose expectations have been met?
- Am I comfortable with telling other counsellors or my supervisor what I am considering doing?

These are all questions that can be considered in supervision or with experienced colleagues. The aim is not to imply that only the client ought to benefit and everything is a sacrifice by the counsellor in the interests of the client. It is ethically acceptable for a counsellor to benefit from offering counselling by getting a fair reward and personal satisfaction. The difficulties arise when a client is no longer the first concern in the counselling and has become secondary to meeting the counsellor's needs or interests.

Curiously one of the situations in which clients may be particularly vulnerable to exploitation arises during training. Trainees are often under pressure to demonstrate their proficiency within quite tight time limits determined by the training programme. The level of investment of themselves financially and the sense of vulnerability when being assessed can combine, with the result that trainees put their own needs ahead of those of their clients. A client who is progressing well or seems likely to do so is a very tempting subject for a case study or a recording to demonstrate practice skills. How much pressure ought the client be put under to take part in generating material for the counsellor's training and assessment?

Avoiding exploitation of clients

Anne needs a video of her for her training and assessment on a professional counselling course. Frances is just right as a client. How far ought Anne to go in putting pressure on her to be recorded? What ought to be the limits of persuading or pressurizing Anne? What should she do to make sure that her request is ethical? What are the risks if she gets it wrong?

If we ask the powerful questions to expose any exploitation here, then we will discover that there are considerable benefits to counsellors in having material to submit for assessment and the rewards of a qualification if the work passes. Does this make it exploitation? Not necessarily. It is worth asking searching questions about the benefits to the client and the process by which that person has become involved in the assessment process. We can ask the following:

- Have clients been asked to participate in an open-ended and honest way that talks about the implications for them?
- Have clients been informed that whether they accept or decline this will make no difference to the type of service they receive, and certainly not put them at any disadvantage in decisions about what will be best for them?
- What are the implications for confidentiality and how will these be managed?
- What are the safeguards in place to ensure that clients receive the best possible service?
- Have clients been given sufficient explanation of what will be involved and time to reflect on whether or not to take part? Have they given consent that is adequately informed and been given freely?

Clients may often want to please their counsellor for conscious or unconscious reasons. They may hope to strengthen the relationship, be acknowledged as special, have strong feelings of gratitude or any of many possible reasons. These reasons do not of themselves make any client's involvement exploitative if that client also receives significant benefit from the work and the process of involving them has been managed respectfully.

Courses have a large ethical responsibility. They can support their trainees in making such requests well and respectfully and model similar respect for their trainees. Alternatively, they can pressurize their students to override any concerns about exploitation and sow the seeds for future insensitivity to clients' interests and their exploitation. Professional pressures can be as dangerous as the more obvious pursuit of the personal, ideological, financial, sexual, and emotional needs of the counsellor.

Responding to Exploitation by Counsellors

Exploitation involves meeting the counsellor's needs or someone else's at the expense of the client's. Exploitation may be deliberate or unintentional, but it is always unethical. What should a counsellor do when they suspect another counsellor of exploiting clients? Their course of action must depend on the circumstances in which the suspicions arise if the client is not to be subjected to further harm.

Marjorie seeks counselling because she feels troubled by her experience with her previous counsellor. She had been having a sexual relationship with her counsellor, which had started while she was receiving counselling. She is aware that this is a breach of the counsellor's code of ethics but does not wish to make a complaint.

In these circumstances the counsellor ought to be bound by his agreement with Marjorie about confidentiality and can only act with her consent. He may actively seek this consent or encourage Marjorie to pursue her own complaint, but if he does more than this he will inevitably compromise his own relationship with his client by failing to work within an agreement about confidentiality and respect her autonomy. Even though the counsellor may feel uncomfortable with this knowledge there is little else he can do; otherwise he will compound the original harm by increasing his client's vulnerability by a further breach of confidence. Marjorie's needs ought to have priority.

What if the client reveals in confidence a situation where a counsellor is repeatedly exploiting many clients? It will then be a matter of judgment whether it would be better to respect an agreement with an individual client about confidentiality or whether it would be better to report the situation in order to prevent further harm to other clients. The significance of considerations of acting to promote the 'public good' with regard to confidentiality is considered in Chapter 10. This is an extremely difficult situation because there can be no hard-and-fast guidelines. Each person has to assess the situation according to the known circumstances. However, it is increasingly accepted that confidential disclosures to the people or bodies able to detect or prevent exploitation or protect client safety that have been made in good faith will usually be ethically and legally justified. Client safety will usually override confidentiality.

Sandy, a counsellor and colleague, tells you confidentially that he has started a sexual relationship with a current client.

In this alternative situation there is a crucial difference: the counsellor, not the client, has approached you directly. Notwithstanding the agreement about confidentiality, it is probably better to encourage Sandy to report the circumstances to his professional association and seek their guidance and, if this does not happen, to take the initiative yourself. A counsellor who actively seeks assistance for himself is likely to be viewed more favourably than someone who waits to be reported. However, even in this situation, because the counsellor has approached you in confidence, there should be no automatic breach of confidence. Again, it is a matter of weighing up whether you are more likely to promote the 'public good' by breaking a confidence or by keeping that confidence. This constraint does not operate if you are told of the sexual relationship without any preconditions relating to confidentiality. Again, client safety will usually override confidentiality.

Sometimes allegations of exploitation will occur as rumour. For example, you were at a party and you heard allegations that a counsellor you know well and have worked with is financially exploiting her clients. There would be some doubt about the credibility of such a rumour because you do not have direct personal evidence. If you think that it is unbelievable, then you may wish to let the counsellor know about the existence of the rumour so that she can choose what to do about it. If the counsellor admits to you that the rumour has an element of truth, you are in a similar position to the second example. If, on the other hand, you have reason to suspect the rumour might be true, but the counsellor denies it, then it is a matter of personal judgment how to proceed or whether to wait and see if your suspicions are confirmed or disproved.

All the major counselling organizations place an obligation on counsellors to challenge any suspected malpractice by other members of that organization and to report the malpractice when this is appropriate. The act of reporting a fellow counsellor can seem extremely daunting and full of potential conflict and embarrassment.

However, these are seldom sufficient reasons for not doing so. Far more important as the basis of your decisions is the appropriate protection of clients' rights and, ultimately, the members of the public who seek counselling.

Conclusion

The exploitation of clients raises important issues for counsellors. It is not merely a matter of harm to the clients most directly concerned but to the reputation of counselling as a whole; these are hard judgments for counsellors to make. Counsellors tend to value diversity in people and relationships. When faced with clear examples of exploitation it is all too easy either to under-react by maintaining an inappropriate level of non-judgmentalism or to over-react with excessive zeal. Neither of these responses is helpful. Exploitative practices must be challenged and eliminated, but as this chapter has shown it requires great care to assess the issues involved in specific situations and to be fair to the client and everyone else involved.

To access the online resources accompanying this chapter, please visit: https://study.sagepub.com/reevesandbond

10

Confidentiality

Chapter Overview

Confidentiality provides the conditions essential to **counselling** that enable clients to talk freely. This chapter explores the ethical basis of confidentiality with a detailed consideration of the obligations and exceptions to observing confidentiality. It concludes by examining whether clients should be expected to observe confidentiality and the **ethics** of collaboration between professionals.

Key words

confidentiality, **privacy**, **disclosure**, **public interest**, collaboration

Confidentiality is probably the issue that raises the most ethical and legal anxiety for counsellors. It is one over which practice has evolved from a total commitment to a client's **privacy** and confidentiality to something that requires active management by the counsellor and may involve making difficult judgments. These changes have taken place in response to a greater appreciation of the ethical complexities of providing **counselling**, but also have been driven by changes in the **law**.

The Importance of Confidentiality in Counselling

Confidentiality is considered fundamental to counselling because by its very nature counselling is an intimate relationship which often involves the client in divulging information about their current and past situations as well as their opinions and innermost feelings (Mitchels and Bond, 2021). This can only take place in a relationship based on **trust**. In particular, a client needs to feel that whatever has been disclosed will not be used in ways that will harm them. This usually means that **disclosures** in counselling are made by clients on the assumption that what is said remains confidential between the counsellor and client.

Confidentiality acts as a shield to protect client **autonomy** by putting them in control of how they use their counselling in their everyday life. Confidentiality protects against unwelcome intrusions from the counselling room into other areas of a client's life. It also provides protection against any stigma associated with having sought help (Holmes and Lindley, 1998).

One meaning of confidentiality is 'strong trust' (from the Latin *con-fidere*). High levels of trust are necessary to create the conditions in which clients can strive for the levels of personal truthfulness that are necessary to address the issues that are causing them concern. It requires corresponding levels of trustworthiness on the part of the counsellor. For these reasons, protecting confidentiality is a high ethical priority in counselling and requires sound ethical reasons for confidentiality to be curtailed in any way. However, professional attitudes to confidentiality have changed over time in the face of other competing ethical demands, particularly the protection of vulnerable people and children from harm.

The Historical Commitment to Total Confidentiality

Psychoanalysis has traditionally taken a very robust view of confidentiality and the protection of clients' privacy. Some psychoanalysts have been prepared to risk prison in order to protect confidences. In a remarkable account of being summoned to court to give evidence, Anne Hayman (1965: 786) described how she successfully persuaded a judge to exercise his discretion to allow her not to give evidence. She appeared in court with her own legal representation and presented the following argument for refusing to disclose her patient's confidences even though she had that person's permission to do so:

> Suppose a patient had been in treatment for some time and was going through a temporary phase of admiring and depending upon me; he might therefore feel it necessary to sacrifice himself and give permission, but it might not be proper for me to act on this.

This example involves a vital principle. Some states in the USA have a law prohibiting psychiatrists from giving evidence about a patient without the patient's written permission, but this honourable attempt to protect patients misses the essential point that they may not be aware of unconscious motives impelling them to give permission. It may take months or years to understand things that were said or done during analysis, and until this is achieved it would belie all our knowledge of the workings of the unconscious mind if we treated any attitude arising in the analytic situation as if it were part of an ordinary social interchange. If we allow and help people to say things with the ultimate aim of helping them to understand the real meanings underlying what may well be a temporary attitude engendered by transference, it would be the crassest dishonour and dishonesty to permit unwarranted advantage to be taken of their willingness to avail themselves of the therapeutic situation. It would be as if a physician invited a patient to undress to be examined, and then allowed the law to see them naked and arrest them for exhibiting themself. Where no permission has been given, the rule to maintain discretion is, of course, similarly inviolable. Clients attend counsellors on the implicit understanding that anything they reveal is subject to special protection. Unless a counsellor explicitly states that this is not so, both parties have a tacit agreement, and any betrayal of this only dishonours the counsellor. That the agreement may not be explicit is no excuse. Part of a counsellor's work is to put into words things which are not being said. They are the responsible party in the relationship, so surely it is they who should pay, if there is any price to be paid, because something has not been stated clearly (Hayman, 1965).

What was remarkable about Anne Hayman's level of commitment to absolute confidentiality is that she was prepared to accept the consequences of refusing to give evidence. In the late 1980s, counsellors shared with other members of the psychological therapies an instinctively protective approach to clients' confidences. For example, Einzig (1989), in the first edition of *Counselling and Psychotherapy – Is It for Me?*, a publication designed to inform potential clients, stated that 'all counselling is totally confidential'.

However, there is also some limited evidence from that time that certain services were promising higher levels of confidentiality than they were prepared to deliver. When the Children's Legal Centre conducted a survey of over 100 counselling services for young people, they found that although many initially considered that they were committed to 'total confidentiality many changed their view on further consideration':

> There are some agencies who do guarantee absolute confidentiality (although it is debatable whether some of them, on further questioning, would have acknowledged extreme circumstances in which even they would feel forced to breach confidentiality – what if a child comes in and shows a counsellor a bottle of deadly poison which they intend to pour into the city's water supply …).

> Others had carefully defined exceptional circumstances. But a sizeable number showed a worrying degree of confusion – suggesting in answer to one question that they did guarantee confidentiality, and then proceeding to indicate very wide exceptions (e.g. if a client child was thought to be 'at risk'). (Children's Legal Centre, 1989)

This is at the heart of the ethical problem. How far can a counsellor go in making confidentiality a priority over all other ethical concerns, such as the protection of others from serious harm?

The limits of confidentiality

Liam has benefited greatly from counselling. However, in a passing remark, he reveals something that causes his counsellor to be concerned about the safety of other students and the college buildings. How should the counsellor respond ethically? Where do the limits of confidentiality end and other ethical priorities take over?

Counsellors have not been alone with this ethical dilemma. Finding a way of reconciling conflicting pressures in favour of privacy and confidentiality, while requiring or permitting ethically desirable disclosures of confidences, has been accelerated by developments in the law that are applicable to all citizens. These developments have resulted in both greater legal protection for clients' confidences and greater clarity when breaches of clients' confidences may be required. Current law requires counsellors to make carefully considered judgments as to what would be the best outcome and to be legally accountable for those decisions.

Pause for Reflection

How would you respond in the situation with Liam? How will you manage your conflicting ethical obligations to respect your client's confidences and your concern to protect other people (and the building) from harm?

Legal Protection of Confidentiality

The protection of a client's confidences and privacy is a legal obligation required by several levels of the law. It is only possible to give a broad overview of the law in relation to confidentiality; for a fuller consideration of how the law impacts on practice see Mitchels and Bond, *Confidentiality & Record Keeping in Counselling & Psychotherapy* (2021).

The Human Rights Act 1998 created legal obligations for all 'public authorities' and is therefore directly applicable to all counselling provided in statutory services (e.g. health, education and social services) and indirectly reaches wider than this. Article 8 concerns the protection of privacy and is set out in two parts. The first part establishes the general right to privacy and the second sets out the limits of these **rights**:

> Article 8.1 Everyone has the right to respect for his private and family life, his home, and his correspondence.
>
> Article 8.2 There shall be no interference by a public authority with the exercise of this right except as in accordance with the law and as is necessary in a democratic society in the interests of national security, public safety, or the economic well-being of the country, for the prevention of disorder or crime, for the protection of health or morals, or the rights and freedoms of others.

This sets the right to privacy and confidentiality within the wider social context of the structures required to protect a democratic society. This is the wider legal context that is easily forgotten when sitting in the counselling room with the door closed against the outside world. All the people in the room are citizens and subject to the law which both protects confidences disclosed in that room but may limit that protection.

The Data Protection Act 1998 set out requirements that were applicable across the European Union, and these were further developed in the EU General Data Protection Regulations (GDPR) in 2018, which apply to all EU members. The UK's vote in 2016 to leave the EU and subsequent negotiations opens up the possibility of further changes to data protection that are independent of the EU. However, any changes have considerable impact way beyond counselling, especially for international trade, so that they are likely to be widely debated and consulted upon well in advance of the changes taking effect. It seems very likely that the GDPR will be the legal basis for data protection for the foreseeable future in the UK. As counselling records fall within the category of 'sensitive personal data', they will remain subject to the most stringent requirements for confidentiality and the safe storage of any records.

Common law applies in any circumstances not covered by statute. The obligation to protect information given in confidence is established where the recipient of the information knows or ought to know that the other person can reasonably expect his privacy to be respected (see the case of *A v B plc and C* ('Flitcroft') [2002]). Therefore, it follows that counsellors owe their clients a general legal duty of confidentiality.

Exceptions to a Duty of Confidentiality

There are a number of exceptions to a general legal duty of confidentiality for counsellors. These can arise where the client waives a right to confidentiality by giving their consent to **disclosure**, where the law recognizes a countervailing factor that outweighs a right to confidentiality, or where there is a legal obligation to disclose. The first of these provides a practical basis for involving the client in deciding how to resolve many ethical **dilemmas** over confidentiality:

1. The obligation to protect confidential information ceases if a client (who is the subject of that information) consents to disclosure. Typically, the consent will be to disclose specific information to specified people or organizations or for specific purposes. Going beyond the client's conditions for granting consent will amount to a legal breach of confidence unless there is some other legal justification. Seeking a client's consent to making a disclosure is the best way of overcoming any ethical difficulties. Oral consent is sufficient, but a record of the consent made as close to the time of the consent as possible provides additional protection to client and counsellor in case there is a later disagreement about what the client consented to. This record should include any conditions required by the client that limit their consent to what may be disclosed. A later record of what was disclosed and to whom it was disclosed is further protection and demonstrates ethically and legally informed practice.
2. The balance of **public interest** is probably the most important criterion for overriding confidentiality, especially if this is against the client's wishes or it has not been possible to obtain consent. The counsellor is required to balance the public interest between the public good served by preserving confidentiality and the public good served by breaching confidentiality. The protection of members of the public from serious physical harm would usually tip the balance in favour of disclosure. There are a number of criteria that a counsellor would be wise to consider before breaching confidentiality on a balance of public interests. Mitchels and Bond (2021) recommend consideration of:

   i. *The degree of risk*: a real risk of harm weighs towards breaching confidentiality. A client who has made similar threats but not acted on them would represent a lower risk.
   ii. *The seriousness of the harm being prevented*: the risk of serious physical harm, rape or child abuse would be of sufficient harm to be weighed in favour of breaching confidentiality. The prevention of psychological harm without any associated physical harm would not usually be sufficient for protecting adults. It would require the client's consent.

iii. *Imminence:* time to prevent the harm is running out.
iv. *Effectiveness:* there is a reasonable probability that the breach of confidentiality will prevent the harm.

In order to protect the disclosure from legal action for breach of confidence, any disclosure should be made to someone or an organization capable of preventing the harm, the information disclosed should be restricted to what that person needs to know to prevent the harm, and should be made on an explicitly confidential basis. Making a record of the decision-making process and why it is considered that the balance of public interests favours disclosure is considered good practice here. This might include any professional and legal **guidance** sought to inform the decision where the circumstances permit this. A record of when it was disclosed, to whom, what has been disclosed, how the disclosure was made, and the reasons for the disclosure is also considered good practice (marginal decisions to preserve confidentiality on the balance of public interest are probably also best recorded.)

3. The prevention and detection of serious crime. There is no authoritative definition of serious crime that would justify breach of confidence. The Department of Health guidelines (2010: 9) suggest that this category would include murder, manslaughter, rape, treason, kidnapping, child abuse and other cases where individuals have suffered serious harm. It probably also includes harm to state security, public order and substantial financial crimes. It would not usually include theft, fraud and damage to property where the losses are less substantial.

Legal Obligations to Disclose Confidences

The legal obligations to disclose confidences are:

1. *Court orders*: a counsellor can be ordered to appear as a witness or to provide all **records** concerning named clients to a court (called a *subpoena duces tecum* – an order to 'attend and bring the documents with you'). This is a formal order and should not be confused with requests for information from a solicitor, which can be refused. Solicitors tend to send out standard letters requesting 'all **notes** and records', but they may accept an offer from the therapist of a report instead. This might obviate the need to provide all the records and is a commonly accepted practice by psychologists and psychiatrists. If a report and/or notes are refused, a solicitor may seek a court order where necessary. For further guidance, see Bond and Sandhu, *Therapists in Court: Providing Evidence and Supporting Witnesses* (2005).

2. *Statutory obligations*:
   i. *Terrorism*: there is general duty to report information that assists in the detection or prevention of terrorism and it is a separate offence known as 'tipping off' to give anyone information about the disclosure that might interfere with an investigation (Terrorism Act 2000).
   ii. *Child protection*: counsellors working in statutory services, such as health, children's services and education, may be required to provide information to authorities responsible for the prevention and detection of child abuse. Some counsellors working in non-statutory services may be required to make disclosures through their contract of employment. The level of difficulty encountered by any single professional adequately assessing the degree of risk to a child creates a strong ethical case for conforming to legal obligations under the Children Acts 1989 and 2004 and voluntary co-operation where there is no strict legal obligation to do so. For guidance, see *Working Together to Safeguard Children* (Department for Education, 2018). Following child abuse scandals involving the DJ Jimmy Savile, the entertainer Rolf Harris and the publicist Max Clifford, there are likely to be proposals to revise the law on child protection and revised guidance, although at the time of writing the legal position remains the same.

Child protection cases can be both ethically and personally challenging for counsellors. Good counselling practice shows respect for clients' control and authority over their lives in contrast to their experiences of being abused. Where we are working with adults recalling abuse, counsellors can usually respect their wishes about whether they want to report the person who assaulted them. The victim has the choice about whether or not to report a crime. However, if the adult discloses the identity of the abuser and that they believe that person has access to other children or may be abusing them, then the counsellor may be faced with an acute ethical dilemma. There has been increased pressure on counsellors to report instances of historical abuse (abuse that has allegedly occurred sometime in the past), even when the name of the abuser is not immediately known. The counsellor is faced with a choice between conflicting ethical obligations to respecting client autonomy and confidentiality or acting to protect other children from abuse. It is common for abused clients to be reluctant to become involved in reporting their abuser even to protect others. They have been intimidated and often bullied into submission or groomed with presents and 'being special'. A combination of fear of the abuser and shame is a powerful cocktail that can create a desperate desire for confidentiality. On the other hand, the counsellor may feel an ethical duty (often a legal duty depending on the setting) to act to protect other potential victims.

Pause for Reflection

Can you consider any instances for maintaining client confidentiality where child protection concerns are raised, for example in the event of suspected historical abuse? Or should concerns always be communicated regardless of the client's position?

Child protection and confidentiality

Frank is a young adult who is talking about the impact of having been abused by his step-father. He does not want his step-father to be prosecuted and asks for his confidences to be protected. However, he reveals that his step-father is now living with a younger half-brother, Alfie. He thinks that Alfie is not at risk of abuse by his step-father – but is not sure. Frank feels strongly that he wants his confidences protected. What should his counsellor do – keep his confidences or report abuse for each of these situations to an agency that could investigate and, if necessary, intervene?

Contractual Obligations to Disclose Confidential Information

A breach of confidence would not be justified simply because it was required by a contract of employment. The Law Commission on *Breach of Confidence* (1981) considered a situation that was relevant to counsellors:

> A doctor or a psychologist employed in industry is faced with the demand by his employer for the disclosure of medical records relating to other employees of the firm who have frankly discussed their personal problems with him on a confidential basis and without any express or implied understanding that the information would be made available to the employer.
>
> Assuming that no question of the public interest is involved (as it might be, for instance, if the health or safety of other employees was at stake), we think that the doctor or psychologist must preserve the confidences of those who confide in him. Of course, if he only accepts the confidence on the express or implied understanding that, pursuant to his contractual duty, he may disclose the information to the employer, this would constitute a limitation on the scope of the obligation of confidence to which he is subject.

This guidance requires the counsellor to have sought the client's consent to disclosures that are not a statutory requirement or can be justified on the balance of public interest. Failing to do so places counsellors in a 'Catch-22' situation where they are forced to choose between breaching an obligation of confidentiality or their contract of employment. Whichever way is chosen, this is likely to incur legal penalties and may also result in professional conduct proceedings. Planning ahead to meet all one's legal obligations by ensuring overall compatibility between them and also ensuring that clients are adequately informed about the terms on which counselling is being offered is the only way to avoid these legal difficulties. The employer should be made aware of the deterrent impact of restrictions to confidentiality and the ethical significance of confidentiality in counselling so that all restrictions are purposeful and kept to a minimum.

Suicidal Clients

In UK law there is no general duty to report suicidal risk or serious **self-harm** concerning adults. There is a long tradition that any adult may refuse treatment for physical **illness** for good reasons, irrational reasons, or no reasons. A counsellor is legally obliged to respect the wishes of an adult client with mental capacity who is contemplating **suicide** and actively forbids the counsellor to seek additional help. Public policy in favour of reducing levels of suicide would justify the counsellor in using all their powers of persuasion to avert the suicide or to obtain permission to get additional help. Where mental illness is suspected, it may be appropriate to consult the client's GP (if known), social services or a psychiatric service to see if the client meets the requirements for a compulsory admission to hospital for assessment or treatment under mental health legislation. Where counsellors are working in some statutory services or on behalf of public bodies, there may be a **duty of care** to take reasonable steps to prevent suicide, particularly in residential settings, or it may be included as a duty in the contract of employment. Knowing your agency requirements and making compatible agreements with clients are the best ways of managing legal requirements and any constraints on confidentiality associated with suicide and self-harm (Reeves, 2010, 2015). (See Chapter 7 for a further discussion.)

Where the method of suicide risks serious physical harm to others, for example by jumping off a bridge into traffic or jumping off a building over pedestrians, the balance of public interests would usually favour breach of confidence if the risk is real and imminent.

Children and Young People

The law relating to young people under the age of 18 with life-threatening conditions is more protective of their ongoing survival than that of adults as a matter of public policy. There is a presumption in common law that favours enabling young people to reach adulthood. The balance of public interest (see above) would probably favour breach of confidence to obtain advice or services where there is an imminent risk of suicide or death due to self-harm, especially if there is no other reasonable way of preventing it. Depending on the availability of local services, it may be possible to obtain advice from children's services, child and adolescent mental health units, or voluntary organizations specializing in supporting young people. The practical difficulty facing anyone seeking help and advice is the comparative shortage of services to protect young people from self-harm in contrast to the growth of services to protect young people from abuse and neglect by their carers and others. The imposition of treatment against a valid refusal of consent by a young person or someone with parental responsibility would require either legal authority from mental health legislation or an order from the High Court.

Does the Client Have a Duty of Confidentiality?

It is a common question about whether a client is bound to keep everything that happens in the counselling confidential. Two arguments in favour of expecting clients to observe strict confidentiality are usually offered. First, total secrecy helps to set a boundary between the counselling and the rest of the client's life. The existence of this boundary may increase the intensity of the personal experience of counselling and therefore its effectiveness. It may also prevent interference from partners and friends. Second, counsellors may be quite disclosing about themselves during counselling. This is an issue of particular importance for the users of the person-centred approach and related methods that require a counsellor to be self-revealing.

Although these are strong arguments, the adverse effects of attempting to impose confidentiality on a client may counter them. First, on ethical grounds, it would be limiting the client's control of the outcome of the counselling and would be difficult to enforce without undermining the counselling by putting the counsellor in the conflicting roles of counsellor and enforcer. Second, the issue of confidentiality is complex enough for the counsellor without the need to develop parallel **standards** for the client. Third, most clients have considerable emotional barriers against seeking counselling because of the necessity of acknowledging their own neediness. To impose confidentiality on clients could increase these personal barriers because of a widespread cultural tendency to associate secrecy with shame. Therefore, a general principle of client secrecy seems inappropriate.

Occasionally, it may be appropriate for the counsellor to say something in confidence to a client. Usually this would be because the counsellor is about to say something which is personally sensitive about themself and wishes to retain control of whom they inform. For example, a counsellor with relevant personal experience who is working with a sexually abused client may wish to say something about their own experience of being sexually abused and how they overcame it. The counsellor needs to be aware that any attempt to enforce confidentiality on the client would raise the ethical difficulties already mentioned. Therefore, counsellors do sometimes have to accept that some clients might break confidences and counsellors are unlikely to be able to do much about it. Both client and counsellor take a risk in confiding in each other. Observance of ethical guidelines by counsellors minimizes the risk to clients but counsellors are not protected in the same way. Counsellors need to assess which clients to confide in and recognize that there is some unavoidable risk of that confidence being broken.

In child care cases, the family court can make orders about the retention and confidentiality of documents in the case, which might include therapy reports and records. This power may also apply in some circumstances to certain criminal cases where confidentiality is necessary in the public interest.

Pause for Reflection

Do you ask your clients to keep the session contents confidential? What are the implications of this from your experience in practice?

Collaboration between Professionals

Counsellors are increasingly working in teams or agencies with other counsellors, or in settings like primary care or education where collaboration between professionals with different functions is considered desirable or necessary. Where information is shared on a strictly confidential basis within the boundaries of a team, clients may benefit from:

- minimizing the repetition of what may be a painful history or event being told repeatedly to each member of the team;
- better co-ordination between the people delivering services;
- greater opportunities for service providers to pool knowledge and expertise and enhance the quality of service offered;

- the opportunity to be involved in decisions about which information is shared and with whom. Clients may be deprived of this opportunity where exchanges of information are informal or ad hoc, and thus outside their awareness.

Developments in new technology have extended the possibilities for consultations and discussions between staff and for data-sharing, particularly of computerized records. In 1997 the Caldicott Committee produced a report which recommended six principles for information-sharing in the NHS and between the NHS and non-NHS organizations. The six Caldicott principles are:

1. Justify the purpose(s) for using confidential information.
2. Only use when absolutely necessary.
3. Use the minimum that is required.
4. Access should be on a strict need-to-know basis.
5. Everyone must understand his or her responsibilities.
6. Understand and comply with the law.

The personally sensitive nature of information disclosed in counselling suggests that clients should know what is being shared and with whom and for what purpose, and then have the opportunity to consent to this.

This principle of respecting client autonomy by putting them in control of what is communicated about them should arguably also be applied to information-sharing to conform to professional standards, such as ongoing and regular counselling **supervision** or seeking a client's consent to be presented for training purposes.

There has been one inquiry which considered the responsibility of counsellors working in healthcare teams. This concerned Anthony Smith, who murdered his mother and step-brother while suffering from paranoid schizophrenic delusions. An inquiry into his care was commissioned by Southern Derbyshire Health Authority and Derbyshire County Council (SDHA, 1996). Prior to this tragedy, he had been receiving counselling in his GP's practice and a range of community- and hospital-based psychiatric services. The report considered many different aspects of his treatment and made a large number of recommendations that extended well beyond counselling. With regard to counselling, the report was critical of the caution with which counsellors managed confidentiality. In particular, it argued that there ought to be an ethical obligation to breach confidentiality to the extent of having confidential discussions with other members of the clinical team where the counsellor suspects that a client is becoming seriously mentally ill and poses a threat to themself or others. It also recommended that counsellors should be trained in the recognition of mental illness. These recommendations undoubtedly deserve serious consideration when developing **agency policy** and implementation in ways that are compatible with the Caldicott principles that were published a year later. The general principle that there should be clarity about management of confidentiality and communications between team members is one that merits wide support.

Pause for Reflection

What perspective do you hold with respect to the management of confidentiality, beyond those instances where breaching confidentiality is a legal requirement? Does your approach support the possibility of multidisciplinary working, or inhibit it, and what are the consequences of this for your clients?

Penalties for Breach of Confidence

The remedies and penalties applied indicate the level of seriousness with which courts view breaches of confidence. The court may issue orders (i.e. injunctions) to prevent a proposed disclosure of confidential information. These only work where the person affected has prior notice of an intention to breach confidence. After a breach of confidence has taken place, the court may award damages and this is the most likely outcome, especially if the client is fee-paying. The damages may be substantial if it can be shown that there was damage to social reputation, severe injury to feelings, job loss, reduced prospects of promotion or other losses. Damages may be awarded even if the client has not suffered any economic loss because there may be no better way of acknowledging the harm that has been done. Imprisonment is also a possible outcome. A judge has speculated that imprisonment would be an appropriate penalty for a health worker who leaked the names of doctors with AIDS to the press (*X v Y*, 1988).

Alternative ways for clients to resolve breaches of confidentiality are to seek a Data Protection Compliance Order (or equivalent in other countries where available) if the professional is a data controller, which would usually be the case if the counsellor (alone or jointly) determines the purposes for which the data are processed. A client may also bring a complaint against a counsellor to an employer or any professional body to which that counsellor belongs.

Conclusion

Although the law of confidentiality in the UK and elsewhere is complex, it is frequently compatible with ethical analysis. Confidentiality is a high ethical and practical priority in order to avoid deterring clients from taking up counselling and to create the conditions that make counselling effective. However, confidentiality is a secondary requirement to make primary ethical concerns possible, such as respecting client autonomy, fidelity or honouring trust and doing good and avoiding harm. When understood in this way, confidentiality is not an end in itself, and nor should it be the primary ethical principle to guide all actions.

There are some situations where offering total confidentiality would compromise the integrity of the counsellor. Counsellors may find themselves faced with difficult ethical decisions to protect their own integrity and that of counselling. Where does integrity lie if a client insists on the counsellor respecting their autonomy by maintaining confidentiality in order to enable them to violate someone else's autonomy by causing them serious harm or committing a serious crime against them? Similarly, ought clients to be able to insist that a counsellor remains **trustworthy** by protecting their confidences when a client is being seriously untrustworthy to others by exposing them to serious harm? The law goes a long way to protect confidentiality and establishes criteria by which a counsellor would be expected to justify any breaches of confidentiality. In most situations, it ought to be possible to find a way to reconcile law and ethics.

To access the online resources accompanying this chapter, please visit: https://study.sagepub.com/reevesandbond

11

Counselling Online

Chapter Overview

This chapter reviews the ethical implications of the use of **digital** technologies in **counselling** and as a counsellor more generally, and the distinctive ethical benefits and challenges involved. Issues including **security**, educating clients, relationship **boundaries**, and working across legal jurisdictions are considered.

Key words

internet, digital, hyperspace, **online**, email, social forums, technological **competence**, jurisdiction

The use of **digital** technology and **online** communications has transformed the living and social environment over the last 30 years for everyone who has access to it. People have witnessed a revolution in the speed of communication, with letters replaced by email, expensive international phone calls replaced by Skype and other online audio and video communications, and a proliferation of different applications of **social media** such as Twitter, LinkedIn, Facebook, Instagram, TikTok and so on, and online forums.

While there has been a slow but steady recognition of the value of technology as a mechanism for facilitating therapeutic relationships over the years, the COVID-19 pandemic of 2020 and the world lockdown during the crisis prompted large numbers of counsellors to embrace the technologies, as face-to-face work became impossible. Simply put, they faced either having to make the shift to online work, or not being able to see clients at all, with the obvious detriment to many thousands of clients already engaged in therapy, as well as the financial implications for counsellors, particularly those working in private practice and the third sector, where the subsequent financial crisis hit particularly hard. However, all counsellors had to face quick decisions, as well as major changes in the training of counsellors: students had traditionally obtained their practice hours via face-to-face placements, but this now became impossible. The use of online technology shifted overnight from the margins of counselling to the mainstream.

New technology continues to erode, with its own rapid developments, the significance of national boundaries by making international communication so much easier, and thus changing the context in which lives are lived locally. Distance is no longer the barrier to communications between people that it once was. For an older generation, it is a process of bringing themselves alongside these new developments; for younger people who have grown up alongside this rapidly developing technology, the experience has been very different. The virtual world is not an add-on but is experienced as integral to how they communicate with people. The distinction between the virtual and the real world of face-to-face interaction no longer exists for many young people. Emotional wellbeing and identities are being transformed by interactions online, for good or bad. It also appears that ideas about public and private space appear to be shifting across generations as so much of other people's lives is made visible digitally.

These changes provide a combination of challenges and opportunities for counsellors. There is accumulating evidence from online **counselling** services that the new media make it possible to access sections of the community that were previously hard to reach, through a plethora of online mental health self-support packages in the guise of websites and smartphone apps. Extending the reach of services designed to promote mental wellbeing is highly desirable ethically in terms of enhancing the capacity to do good. Providing services to hard-to-reach groups, particularly those with significant issues and challenges in their lives, enhances our ability to satisfy the principle of **justice**. As with any new development, particularly on this scale and developing so rapidly, there are substantial ethical challenges.

Pause for Reflection

To what extent have you made active use of online support packages with your clients, and do you know what professional benchmarks you draw on to judge whether you consider them to be appropriate or not?

Counsellors' Concerns about Working Online

It is in the nature of digital technology that there is constant change and new developments may be short-lived. To be static is to be superseded in the digital world. Developments triggered by the COVID-19 pandemic have meant that technological innovation has been taking place at great speed, and some platforms considered appropriate for counselling became embroiled in concerns about security. Horror stories were recounted of online training being hacked, with participants being witness to distressing images of pornography. Likewise, however, such accounts further supported the call for greater security; major platform providers realized that security with accessibility was the new requirement, with security updates and platform enhancements being issued on a near-daily basis. The new world order called for proficiency in technology, in delivering therapy via a remote mechanism (telephone, text, email or web camera-based), and for counsellors to learn it all overnight.

Most national professional bodies provide some **guidance** on online counselling. There are also specialist organizations that work at the cutting edge of new developments:

- American Distance Counseling Association
- International Society for Mental Health Online
- Online Counselling and Therapy in Action
- Association for Counselling and Therapy Online (ACTO)

There are also a steadily growing number of useful specialist publications (ACTO, 2020; Anthony and Merz Nagal, 2015; Jones and Stokes 2009; Weinberg and Rolnick, 2019; Weitz, 2014), all with examples of actual practice and suggestions for good practice.

The internet and digital technology cannot be ignored in contemporary counselling practice in developed economies. They have become the medium for routine communications between people. There will be few counsellors – and these in declining numbers – who do not use the internet for some aspects of their work with clients. National lockdown seemed to provide a shared reflective space, with many thinking about life before and how they would change it for the future. Counsellors who had for many years only worked face to face considered remaining online as lockdown restrictions came and went, or to proceed in a 'blended' way, of adopting a greater online presence combined with some face-to-face work. Others of course, preferred to move back into an exclusive face-to-face environment, albeit slowly. Online, however, does not represent just one way of working, as there are number of ways of working virtually. These include:

- *Online synchronous services*: live video counselling sessions, live chat rooms and social forums, and *Second Life* in which both client and counsellor are represented by avatars.
- *Online asynchronous services*: counselling by email correspondence or any method of communication on social media that involves a time delay between sending and responding to messages.
- *Administrative and professional support for counselling services*: setting up and managing appointments, organizing routine communications and monitoring client progress or take-up of services.
- *The provision of supplementary information and self-help activities*: self-assessment forms, links to other related services, online guidance.
- *The use of online social forums*: where users can post messages to which other users can respond in ways that often have parallels with traditional groupwork in terms of sharing experiences and offering mutual support.
- *The use of apps on smartphones*: for clients to log their sleep, changes in mood, energy levels and other features of their emotional lives rather than rely on memory alone.

Each of these services raises distinctive ethical challenges to which can be added the **ethics** of managing the technological basis of the work and the distinctive legal issues.

Social Justice in Context

From a social justice perspective, there are advantages and disadvantages of working online. Providing counselling online offers an opportunity for a greater choice of counsellor as the client is not limited by geographical location. Likewise, the costs of travel to counselling, which for some might be prohibitive, cease to be a consideration. Additionally, it has been argued that online counselling might be a better match for some clients who would otherwise not walk through the door of a counselling agency (e.g. some with particular mental health problems or social phobias). Conversely, however, online counselling requires a safe space at a client's home where counselling can take place in privacy, which might be particularly challenging for clients experiencing violence in the home setting for example, as well as the costs of a fast-enough internet connection and equipment to run the apps required to connect to a counsellor.

Digital Interaction between Counsellors and Clients

From face-to-face to online counselling

The move to significantly greater use of online services demands careful reconsideration of the ethical guidance offered, which has typically been developed in the context of face-to-face work being dominant. We need to take each ethical principle in turn.

Being trustworthy

With clients and colleagues online this is every bit as important as it would be in face-to-face communications. Working online creates opportunities to use web-based applications that enable counsellors to create and exchange content with each other and with the public through blogs, micro-blogs (such as Twitter), professional internet forums, content communities (such as YouTube and Flickr) and social networking sites (such as Facebook, Instagram, TikTok and LinkedIn). How you present yourself online will influence your client's perceptions of your integrity and trustworthiness and may also have implications for their perceptions of other members of counselling and related professions. Many practitioners have talked of the potential for clients to disguise their **identity** or location in ways that would not be professionally acceptable for the counsellor providing the service to do. What is striking about searching online services is how many of them provide the identity of counsellors and information about their professional background and qualifications with a photograph. The accuracy and integrity of this information are probably better protected online because that information is so public and therefore so easily questioned or challenged. Nonetheless, it is the ethical **responsibility** of the counsellor to ensure their accuracy. It is also for the counsellor to take reasonable steps to be **trustworthy** as this is within their direct control, but no one can guarantee that they will be trusted as this depends on the responses of others.

One potential source of mistrust that requires active attention is the responsibility to make any conflicts of interest transparent to potential users; for example, any sponsorship of websites should be made clear, and if not obvious openly declared. Being compliant with data protection requirements is a key component for professional integrity. This includes registration with the Information Commissioner's Office and data protection and GDPR requirements concerning the safeguarding of personally sensitive information. For further details of the legal requirements see Mitchels and Bond (2021) *Confidentiality & Record Keeping in Counselling & Psychotherapy*.

Respect for client autonomy

The speed of many internet-based communications means that it is extraordinarily easy to move from enquiry to direct service provision, but this does not override the importance of ensuring that a client is making informed choices or that the terms on which the service is being provided are clarified and agreed before the work commences or the client incurs liability. There are many good examples on the internet of sites prepared by individuals and organizations that provide essential information about the types of service available, any fees to be charged, and the management of **security** and **confidentiality** (in particular any **limitations** to confidentiality and any other significant terms or conditions). The BACP (2019b) advises that websites ought to include **privacy** policy pages which explain how personal data are processed and stored, the security measures being used, and the circumstances under which those data would be disclosed or shared and with whom. For certainty, current best practice and legal position can be checked at the Information Commissioner's Office website (https://ico.org.uk). Clear contracting is as important online as it would be face to face. The parallels between contracting around synchronous sessions online and in the physical world are obvious. More thought is required about asynchronous communications like email (e.g. about agreeing the time limits for the counsellor to reply and how any charges for reading and replying to emails will apply).

Two aspects of counselling ethics are important strategies for protecting client autonomy. These relate to the management of confidential information about clients and the management of dual or multiple relationships. The challenge for confidentiality and privacy is that information online, unless adequately protected, is much more widely available than physically based information. It has potentially unlimited circulation, is easily found by electronic searches, and is extraordinarily difficult or impossible to remove from cyberspace. Again, the counsellor is ethically responsible for the adequate security of their technology and for providing information to clients about how to adequately protect their privacy and confidentiality online. Clients are vulnerable to having their communications intercepted, observed or interfered with unless they take adequate precautions. Their use of work computers, internet cafés or public Wi-Fi compromises their security. Some practitioners provide links to websites that advise on how to manage search histories, adjust privacy settings or other issues that enhance client safety.

The management of dual and multiple relationships in ways that are consistent with the purpose of counselling is as important online as in real life, as risks can arise in both directions. There is nothing to stop clients searching for online information about their counsellors, and nor would it be reasonable to attempt to prevent this and frustrate one of the strengths of the new media which is their transparency and ease of accessibility to all. However, this ought not to prevent counsellors having an online personal life that is independent of their work. Two main strategies are currently widely used to ensure a counsellor's separation of personal and professional online presence: the first is being attentive to the privacy settings of any social media used for personal reasons, and for some the use of a different online identity for personal communications; the second is establishing clear expectations around whether or not a counsellor will accept invitations to be a 'friend' on sites like Facebook, and what will happen should counsellor and client accidentally encounter each other online outside the counselling relationship. Other potential complications arising from client behaviour online can include:

- clients posting communications between themselves and counsellors online;
- clients posting comments on their counsellor's website or blog (probably a more sensitive issue if the remarks are negative or critical).

Doing good and avoiding harm

Many of the strategies involved in being trustworthy and respecting client autonomy will also help to maximize the good and minimize the harm. The major positive contribution made by working online is the increased accessibility of services to people who might find face-to-face work too intimidating or unappealing. For others, online services avoid travelling for counselling, which can be a major obstacle because of the distance, cost, or the physical demands of travelling. The significant harms that can arise from working online relate to the potential for fraud and the potential ease for some people to provide services of inadequate quality. Registration, membership of professional bodies and quality assurance schemes are possibly even more necessary online than would be the case with face-to-face work.

Experience of offering online services is generally positive. It does appear to be just as possible to form therapeutic alliances with clients as it would be in face-to-face working. However, most experienced counsellors recommend undertaking an initial assessment of clients to ensure their suitability for online work. It is widely considered that people with moderate to severe mental **illness** involving psychosis are unsuitable for online counselling. People with alcohol- or drug-related problems may also be better counselled face to face as levels of intoxication are more easily and reliably assessed by direct observation.

Responding to clients in crisis during or between online sessions can be more challenging, particularly when there is considerable geographical distance between counsellor and client. The counsellor is unlikely to know what local services might be available even if the location of the client has been accurately disclosed. The BACP's (2019b: 9) *Working Online in the Counselling Professions* factsheet recommends that:

> Careful consideration ought to be given to how the practitioner will respond to clients who become so distressed or disturbed that they require additional services or support from healthcare providers or their social network. Good practice requires that practitioners are clear from the outset of working with clients about the boundaries between what is provided by their service directly, how any additional support will be sought in emergency situations by the practitioner, and what depends on clients acting on their own initiative. Online resources or guidance may be provided to assist clients in finding appropriate emergency services, especially where clients are communicating from a distance or it is inappropriate or impractical for the practitioner to seek additional services on behalf of their clients.

Justice

Justice involves fair distribution of the available resources and is never more important than when demand exceeds supply. This is particularly relevant to mental health and wellbeing services where all people experience fluctuations of mood throughout their life and a significant minority will experience diagnosable mental illness. Online counselling increases the potential for responding to these situations with the least intrusive intervention that is appropriate to clients' needs. Such stepped care means that available counselling resources can be provided as efficiently as possible, thereby maximizing their reach to as many people as possible.

Self-respect

One of the consequences of working online is that many more of the communications between counsellor and client are recorded in one format or another, and are therefore more available for systematic reflection than in ordinary face-to-face work. Many of these challenges are identical to providing counselling offline but with an additional technological twist. Counsellors working for extended periods sitting in front of monitors may want to take adequate precautions to protect their physical health and wellbeing by ensuring adequate breaks and appropriate postural support.

Online Administrative and Professional Support for Counselling Services

Security is as important for support services as it would be for the direct service to clients. Without adequate protection they are potentially vulnerable to unauthorized intrusion or corruption by electronic viruses and malware. Most of these services will require registration with the Information Commissioner's Office, which provides a useful self-assessment tool within their 'frequently asked questions for enquirers' to check whether registration is necessary. Transcription of sessions and all other hard copy **records** require the same level of security as records for face-to-face counselling.

The Provision of Supplementary Information and Self-help Activities

Many counselling services with responsibilities for defined communities, such as students, employees or others, are making increasing use of online self-help programmes. Such programmes have been endorsed by NICE as suitable interventions for mild to moderate anxiety and depression with a full and up-to-date list available via the NHS website (Mental Health Apps NHS, 2020). As a consequence, self-help has become a substantial part of low-intensity interventions in Improving Access to Psychological Therapies (IAPT). There is an ethical responsibility on the person who posts self-help guidance to ensure that this is up to date and of adequate quality. In his useful appraisal of internet self-help, Stewart (2014) provided a set of criteria for measuring website quality, including:

- *Accountability* by the use of the Silberg Scale, which includes whether authors and affiliations are identified, if sources and references have been given, the **disclosure** of website ownership, sponsorship or advertising, and up-to-dateness/currency by the disclosure of modification dates. Level of evidence may be determined by the extent to which the help conforms to evidence-based practice.
- *Readability* can be assessed by a number of internet-based tools, including the Flesch-Kincaid Grade Level score which relates to USA school grades so that the lower the score the greater the ease of reading. Personally, we prefer the SMOG readability test widely used in adult education, but there are many others available online.

- *Quality* of information about intervention choice, which can be assessed by six questions from Brief DISCERN that can be found on the internet.
- *Generosity* assessed by willingness to give away resources for free.

These criteria can be used systematically in **research** to produce quantifiable comparative ratings of internet-based self-help, or less precisely to help identify the issues to consider when assessing the quality of potential self-help. The ultimate test is the client experience, and there is some evidence that 'guided' self-help supported by a practitioner is more effective than self-help alone (Gellatly et al., 2007).

The Use of Online Social Forums

There are two major ethical considerations in providing forums for clients and the first relates to client security and respect for their confidentiality and privacy. BACP (2019b) recommends that forum communications should be password protected, that any supplementary email communications to forum users ought not to be identifiable as being from the counsellor or the service provider, and that service users' identities ought to be hidden from other users, possibly by the use of a preferred username.

Best practice suggests that interactions between users on the forum should be supported by house rules designed to create positive norms. Togetherall (https://togetherall.com/en-gb/house-rules, formerly the Big White Wall) offers a number of positive guidelines for behaviour on the forum. To summarize, they include:

- taking responsibility for one's safety;
- protecting one's anonymity;
- asking for support;
- reporting any concerns about abusive behaviour or the safety of others, including the risk of **self-harm**;
- being oneself.

The norms prohibit:

- SHOUTing (the use of capital letters is considered the equivalent to shouting on the internet), bullying, abusing others or acting illegally;
- acting in sexually inappropriate ways or posting pornography;
- impersonating others, whether real or fictional people;
- impersonating people with responsibility for the services.

The use of moderators (people who monitor postings for appropriateness) suggests that offering a forum to the public is a substantial commitment and ought not to be undertaken lightly, and is almost certainly not suitable for counsellors working alone or without the possibility of sharing responsibility for moderating a forum.

Technological Competence

Ensuring a reliable and safe platform is a very basic ethical requirement. An unreliable platform for delivering counselling services is deeply frustrating for clients and often every bit as frustrating as having an unreliable or erratic counsellor. The disruption to therapeutic work is identical. This means that counsellors working online ought to consider their training needs to manage and communicate effectively within their chosen media; this fact came into sharp focus during the COVID-19 pandemic when many counsellors had to upskill their knowledge very quickly. It is also advisable to have either arranged specialist technical support, bound by a contractual commitment to confidentiality, or to subscribe to one of the growing number of secure counselling platforms.

There is always a choice to be made between accessibility to clients and the security of communications. Practitioners hold divided views about the suitability of video conferencing platforms for communicating with clients, such as Skype, Zoom, Microsoft Teams or similar providers. The concern is the uncertain security of such sites. Additionally, the General Medical Council (2013a) advises doctors that 'social media sites cannot guarantee confidentiality whatever privacy settings are in place.' Furthermore, a lot of contextual information can be embedded in photographs, such as location and date. Even deleted material can be recovered. Once material is posted online it takes on a life of its own and on occasions personal information has attracted the attention of the media, been used against employees, or deployed by clients to stalk their counsellors.

There is a strong ethical responsibility for any provider of counselling services online to ensure that these services are managed competently and with sufficient security to meet their clients' needs and their professional ethical requirements.

Jurisdiction and Legal Issues

Although the internet has made it very easy to cross national boundaries, this opportunity has created a number of legal uncertainties and raised other issues:

- When working across national boundaries, there are potentially two legal systems in play (i.e. the counsellor's and the client's). Each may have different legal requirements, so which system applies? This is a troublesome problem shared by all commercial work across national boundaries. There are ongoing attempts to resolve this issue for contracts that operate within Europe. There is no wholly reliable way of controlling the risks of working across different legal jurisdictions, so one widely used solution is to include within the **contract** an explicit statement that the contract is compliant with the laws of England and Wales, for example, and that any disputes will be resolved by the High Courts in London.
- Offering online counselling services to areas where the counselling profession is regulated by national or state law may be illegal. Typically, the legislation that regulates counselling will do so by forbidding the use of a specific professional title by anyone who is not registered within that country or state. This is particularly significant in the USA where counselling is now a regulated profession in all but a very few states. Some counsellors are sufficiently concerned about this legal risk that they have either renamed their services to avoid infringing any protection of title (e.g. by using 'guidance' rather than 'counselling') or refused to take clients who reside in the USA or anywhere else where there is statutory regulation.
- Professional indemnity **insurance** may include working online within the same territory; it does not automatically cover working internationally online. It is important to check with your insurance provider in order to obtain a suitable policy. Even if your contract states that any legal disputes will be resolved according to the law applicable to the counsellor's location, this would probably only apply to contractual disputes. Contractual agreements cannot usually prevent clients from starting actions for civil wrongs (torts), such as **negligence**, in their own country. In some case this may not only be easier to bring a successful case but also may lead to a larger award of damages than would be available in the counsellor's country. Adequate insurance helps to manage this risk.
- Careful thought needs to be given in advance to how you will respond to requests from clients for access to their records or for legal orders to disclose records to courts or the authorities in other countries. In most jurisdictions, clients are legally entitled to access any records kept specifically about them. Disclosure of records both to clients and the authorities is a matter that is best included within the client contract (Chapter 15).

Online for All?

The range of ethical issues involved in providing counselling in cyberspace seems to expand over time as new issues are identified; however, the same ethical principles apply online as would be the case in the physical world. It is the practice of how these principles are applied that may be different. Some believe that there are no ethical issues online for which there are not technological solutions. Others might think this is too optimistic, but that the way the counsellor anticipates ethical issues in order to prevent them becoming problematic is the critical difference.

To access the online resources accompanying this chapter, please visit: https://study.sagepub.com/reevesandbond

12

Working with Social Diversity

Chapter Overview

The ease of travel and the continued proliferation of **digital** technology have increased counsellors' exposure to social **diversity** and **cultural differences** on an unprecedented scale. This chapter considers the ethical implications of **counselling** across many types of differences between counsellor and client. It explores the obligation to be non-discriminatory as ethically necessary but insufficient. The chapter then continues to examine the **ethics** of counselling across cultural differences before considering the importance of cultural **competence**.

Key words

diversity, difference, anti-discrimination, non-discrimination, **tolerance**, **acceptance**, **culture**, cultural competence

Is There a Duty to Counsel across Differences between People?

When a counsellor is working with people who are significantly different from them, either in important characteristics or in social background, the therapeutic challenge involves being able to understand the significance of understanding unfamiliar points of reference in order to make the imaginative leap into someone else's experience in ways that are meaningful to them. This imaginative leap needs to be adequately supported by knowledge that makes real communication possible across differences.

There are two major ethical hazards to be overcome in working across human differences. These hazards are probably intensified by our professional **culture** and assumptions as counsellors. It is a characteristic of most approaches to **counselling** to focus attention on the individual and probably underestimate the significance of the community and social interactions for the client. One of the consequences of this is to be over-reliant on interpreting differences as characteristics of the individual client rather than their social background, community or culture. In the context of a therapeutic relationship, it is often possible to pathologize differences as dysfunctional aspects of a client's personality rather than recognize that their difference may be the result of a counsellor's lack of understanding and reflection. This is the hazard that arises from a too-individualistic approach to people that divorces them from their wider context.

An alternative but equally problematic response to differences between people is to focus on those differences as being characteristic of a wider community in ways that prevent the counsellor engaging with the client as an individual. The obvious examples of this occur where we find ourselves making sweeping statements about the characteristics of another ethnic, national or cultural group. This type of stereotyping can frustrate serious engagement with a client's experience, so that the client is left feeling misunderstood or disrespected. This may not be a counsellor's conscious intention, but the effect on the client is as potentially damaging whether it is conscious or unconscious. A more extreme version of blaming people for their differences is 'scapegoating'. The scapegoat is blamed for what is thought to be wrong with their community and punished (Cousins, 2019).

Social Justice in Context

Recent cases in the USA and elsewhere of institutional racial discrimination and racial violence towards the African American community, including the death of George Floyd in 2020 while being arrested, led to an international movement – #BlackLivesMatter – and widespread protest and anger. The justified reflection that followed prompted many to question what they considered to be embedded racism in the form of monuments glorifying racist actions of the past, including the wealth garnered during the slave trade, and other aspects of racism that had become normalized in mainstream life.

The tearing down of statues triggered a debate about the deconstruction of a culture based on racism, versus the importance of retaining them as a reminder of a racist past. Whatever the relative merits of each position, there was widespread acknowledgement of the importance of engaging with individual and societal reflection on how discriminatory behaviours and beliefs – in this instance around racism, but importantly applicable to all discriminatory behaviours – should be engaged with as a process of genuine, meaningful and sustained change.

The increased mobility of people between communities and around the world and the increasing connectedness through digital mechanisms means that counsellors are increasingly likely to be working with clients from unfamiliar backgrounds. The main ethical strategy for working with differences between people has been a prohibition on **discrimination** (Lago and Smith, 2010). We will consider the application of anti-discriminatory policies in counselling **ethics** before going on to look at the significance of ethical differences between communities and the ways that degrees of difference may require different strategies to make ethical counselling possible. The main definitions for social diversity are given in Figure 12.1.

Equality

Where every person has equal rights and a fair chance. It is an approach where there is recognition that different people have different starting points.

Diversity

'Diverse' means varied or different. We are all different from each other so diversity includes us all. The concept of diversity encompasses acceptance and respect. It means recognizing that each individual is unique and understanding the differences within that person's background.

Inclusion

Where every person feels respected, valued, and that they have a contribution to make.

FIGURE 12.1 *Key definitions for social diversity*

The ethical concern to treat people equally and without discrimination is a characteristic of many contemporary societies. The social and political aims are to produce societies that are cohesive and resilient whilst encompassing sufficient **diversity** to be strongly connected to the rest of the world. Societies that are in conflict or civil war across differences within their communities pay a heavy price in quality of life and the wellbeing of their citizens. As a consequence, many countries have adopted legally enforceable protections against discrimination and the **law** acts as a form of enforceable public morality. This means that counsellors are not unique in their concerns about the damage that discrimination inflicts on people's wellbeing. Rather, these concerns are widely, if unevenly, shared within the communities and organizations in which counsellors work.

The Equality Act 2010 (applicable to England and Wales and adopted by Scotland) provides legal protection against discrimination for specified human characteristics, namely:

- age;
- disability;
- gender reassignment;
- marriage and civil partnership;
- race;
- religion or belief;
- sex;
- sexual orientation.

These protected characteristics are now widely incorporated into the ethical requirements of most professions. Even where this is not the case, the law overrules professional ethics and commercial practice in order to protect people from discrimination.

Recent changes towards the recognition of same sex relationships on the same basis as heterosexual relationships have resulted in legal cases on both sides of the Atlantic. In the UK, traditional Christians, who believed in the importance of marriage as the union of one man and one woman, refused to allow two men who were civil partners to stay in a double room in their bed and breakfast business run in their own home. They took the view that they were entitled to live according to their own **values** under their own roof. The Supreme Court held that discrimination had occurred and awarded damages to the civil partners. A similar difference of view between traditional Christians and a more inclusive attitude to human differences also resulted in a court case in the USA. In *Ward v Wilbanks*, the American Counseling Association provided expert evidence about the ethics of their association. The ACA *Code of Ethics* at that time (ACA, 2005, now 2014) stated that 'Association members recognize diversity and embrace a cross-cultural approach in support of the worth, dignity, potential and uniqueness of people within their social and cultural context.' The district court ruled against a trainee counselling student who had refused to accept a referral of a client who wanted help with feelings of depression and issues related to a same-sex relationship. The Eastern District Court of Michigan found that the university was correct in failing the student because of a serious violation of the ACA *Code of Ethics*. Kaplan (2014: 146), who provided the expert evidence on behalf of ACA, concluded that:

- Professional counselors may not deny counseling services to a homosexual person (or an individual belonging to any other protected class of clients) on the basis of the counselor's values.
- Referrals are to be made on the basis of skill-based competency, not values.
- To avoid abandonment, referral is an option of last resort.
- The counselor's ethical obligation to an individual starts at first contact for assignment not at the first session.

It is a characteristic of discrimination cases that a decision has to be made between conflicting deeply held **rights**. The trend on both sides of the Atlantic and in many other countries has been to find in favour of the most inclusive resolution for all aspects of public life.

The ethical question, which has challenged professional counselling associations, is whether the legally protected characteristics are sufficiently inclusive. For example, the UK Council for Psychotherapy extended in 2009 their commitment to non-discrimination beyond the legally protected categories to include colour, social, economic or immigration status, and lifestyle.

The potential characteristics that can provide discrimination are much wider than those currently covered by legal protection in the UK. Counsellors frequently see how experience of discrimination can undermine someone's confidence or willingness to form relationships with people outside their 'social group'. This can then lead to significant ethical and therapeutic challenges in counselling. For example, in contemporary culture, money represents so much more than having enough to live on and is associated with success and social status. An impoverished client may feel very apprehensive about how a seemingly wealthier counsellor can help them or **respect** them as people. The counsellor needs the communication skills and empathy to overcome the social differences between them. Cultural **competence** is not only about having the knowledge and skills to negotiate major **cultural differences** but also those based on differences in sub-culture shared by counsellor and client.

Pause for Reflection

What do you consider to be your 'defining characteristics' that would be important for another person to understand about you? What makes these characteristics important for you; how do you feel when these are acknowledged, or disregarded, by others?

Trust and ethical mindfulness

Ed is streetwise and has learnt to survive with little money. He is seeking counselling for personal and relationship problems with Jessie that are made worse by poverty. He is finding it hard to trust a counsellor who seems wealthier and more socially privileged than him. How ought his counsellor to respond to the social divide between them? What are her choices?

Most counsellors appear to accept a commitment to being non-discriminatory in their work with clients as a necessary feature of their work. Counselling involves setting aside personal interests in order to assist another person in what they need or want. Being non-discriminatory is therefore necessary but raises the question, 'Is it sufficient?' (Cousins, 2019). There is a qualitative difference in relationships based on **tolerance** from those based on **acceptance**. Tolerance accepts the right of people to be different but does not require active engagement. Acceptance, on the other hand, suggests a closer relationship based on respecting the validity of the other person's differences. This means striving to understand both what matters to the other person in their own circumstances and how that relates to our own.

Counselling across Differences between Cultures

The wheel of human culture and history turns like a kaleidoscope and their interaction produces seemingly unlimited possibilities. Each encounter between people across cultural differences is like a detail in a shifting kaleidoscope of colour and patterns. It is the fluidity and complexity of this subject that makes writing about it in any way that does it **justice** so difficult. McLeod (1997) makes a distinction between traditional, modern and postmodern cultures and their essential characteristics, which can be helpful in understanding the different ethical approaches adopted between cultures but that may also co-exist within cultures. Table 12.1 sets out some of the key characteristics of different cultures.

TABLE 12.1 *Cultural characteristics*

	Traditional	Modern	Postmodern
Ethical focus	Family-focused, collective	Individualistic	Relational
Identity	Self is socially defined: importance of 'honour'	Autonomous, bounded self: importance of 'dignity'	Multi-faceted/split self: importance of quality of relationship

	Traditional	Modern	Postmodern
Faith	Belief in religion	Belief in science	Belief in social construction of knowledge
Moral stance	Moral certainty	Moral relativism	Search for moral framework
Moral purpose	Unchanging society	Commitment to progress	Avoidance of anarchy and chaos
Site of knowledge	Localized forms of political control	Nation state	'Global village'
Typical work	Agricultural work	Industrial work	Information processing

Source: McLeod (1997)

Historically, the shift from traditional to modern cultures probably started in Europe in the early 18th century, with postmodern cultures co-existing with modernity from the late 20th century. In most European communities we can find evidence of the co-existence of these different cultural positions. For example, the conflicts between traditional Christians and tolerance of human differences in sexuality can be viewed as evidence of the transition from a traditional culture, based on long-established religious beliefs, to a late or postmodern tolerance of social diversity made possible by the processes of a modern nation state. These cultural differences are embedded within people's identities and sometimes explain why counselling strategies that are effective with some clients seem to fail so spectacularly with others.

An appreciation of cultural differences and their impact on identity explains why counselling, as developed within the European and North American traditions, often requires considerable modification in order to be useful within other cultures. Although examples of people reflecting on their own experience can be found before the 20th century, it is only in late modern and postmodern times that self-reflection and reflexivity (Giddens, 1991) became a primary purpose of some story narratives. Modern counselling practice is based upon valuing this type of reflexivity for finding meaning, healing and personal development. This is a culturally specific approach that struggles to meet the needs of many people from traditional cultures in Africa and Asia. In cultures that are more action-orientated or hierarchical there may be no tradition of using reflexivity. Authoritative or expert **advice** may be more greatly valued than being supported to think reflexively by a counsellor.

For example, some cultures may understand and express emotions through physical symptoms and, at least initially, show great reluctance to look beyond ill-defined aches and pains to talk about an emotional state of feeling dispirited or depressed. This reluctance may not be solely due to the cultural tools of language and concepts acquired within a particular culture but may also come from the ways in which culture shapes expectations about how people are positioned within society.

One Size Fits All in European Ethics?

There appear to be distinctive cultural differences in how ethical issues affect the talking therapies in different parts of Europe. In northern Europe, and particularly the Scandinavian countries, some viewed the prioritization of respect for the individual that is characteristic of British ethics as quite problematic. In that region the ethical priority would be better characterized as social welfare (i.e. the good of the whole community took precedent over the individual). For example, Sweden was exceptional within Europe in its responses to people affected by HIV or Aids. Drug addicts and sex workers with HIV were imprisoned so that they could be kept under the supervision of medics and psychologists. In 1987, a mental health hospital was converted into a facility for other categories of people considered likely to transmit HIV, especially gay men. A pre-existing system of temporary quarantine for treatable sexually transmissible diseases had become indefinite segregation for what was then considered to be an incurable or untreatable condition. It was, therefore, not surprising that many people who considered themselves to be potentially infected with HIV sought testing in Denmark, which had adopted a different approach to balancing the welfare of society and the rights of the individual.

Counsellors in Greece talked of previous practices of isolating someone who was dying in hospital from other patients, friends and relatives in order to protect those people from the distress of observing a patient's decline and death. In both the Swedish and Greek examples, counsellors spoke of the suffering and fear inflicted on patients and those close to them, no matter how well intentioned the practice. From an ethical perspective, these practices only made sense within an ethical system that prioritized the welfare of the community over that of the individual.

In southern Europe, the application of professional ethics pointed to a different prioritization. An Italian psychologist spoke of the difficulties he had encountered after successfully counselling a suicidal client by using music therapy. In this cultural context, his work was regulated by a deontological code which set out strict expectations of his profession. These required that he should have sought a psychiatric assessment of his client and operated within the prescribed treatment. Even though his experimental use of music therapy had been successful, he was suspended from practising as a psychologist. It appeared that he was working within the context of prioritizing the individual welfare of patients and clients over the **autonomy** of his client, who had chosen him to work outside the usual practices.

TABLE 12.2 *Depiction of ethical discourses*

	Autonomy	Trustworthiness	Individual welfare	Social welfare
Ethical focus	Client/ patient	Client/ practitioner	Client/patient	Society
Decision maker	Patient	Joint	Doctor	1 Doctor 2 Central planning
Primary principle	Autonomy	Being trustworthy	Doing good	Justice
Secondary principle	Doing good	Doing good	Autonomy	Doing good
Consent required	Explicit	Explicit/implicit	Explicit/implicit	Qualified explicit
Test for consent	Reasonable client	Reasonable client	Dutiful counsellor	Dutiful counsellor
Test for negligence	Reasonable patient	Reasonable doctor	Dutiful counsellor	Dutiful counsellor
Right to euthanasia	Yes	Qualified no (double effect)	No*	
Right to abortion	Yes	Qualified yes	No*	Qualified yes
Duty to protect from self-harm/ suicide	Low	Low	High*	High*
Duty to protect others from harm	Qualified low	Qualified low	Medium/high	High

Notes:

* Where a welfare ethic is adopted in association with an ethic in favour of the preservation of human life

Practitioner = anyone providing services relating to physical or mental health, e.g. a counsellor, doctor, nurse, psychologist

In western Europe, it was possible to identify two closely related ethical systems. In one, the patient or client exercises considerable control over the selection of treatments and whether or not to have any treatment at all. For example, in the Netherlands someone who is seriously psychologically distressed can be compulsorily admitted to psychiatric hospital but retains the right to refuse both physical and psychiatric treatments. In the UK, someone with a comparable psychiatric disturbance could be compelled to be a patient in a psychiatric hospital and to receive psychiatric treatment. No matter how irrational or unreasonable that patient's refusal to receive physical treatments appears to be, they retain the right to refuse physical treatment even if it would be life saving. In a famous case, a patient in Broadmoor refused an apparently life-saving operation for gangrene because the voices in his head were telling him to do so. The court upheld his right to refuse the proposed amputation and as a consequence the doctors were required to find alternative treatments that were more acceptable to the voices in his head. In the UK the ethic of respect for the right of adults to control what happens to their body has its roots in Magna Carta (1215). The ethic of respect for the individual's right to self-government, namely autonomy, is almost certainly rooted in the individualism of Protestant beliefs following the Reformation.

An ethic of respect for individual autonomy may seem to be more attractive than the professional ethic of benign paternalism that put all the power in the hands of the professionals to decide what is best for their clients or patients that was characteristic of much mental and physical healthcare until the 1980s. However, one of the limitations of overplaying respect for individual autonomy is practitioners' potential to underestimate their responsibilities for the wellbeing of patients and clients. Many of the health and social care scandals that have been characteristic of the past 50 years are arguably a consequence of professionals failing to fully accept their responsibilities in the partnership between clients and themselves. As a consequence, there has been a renewed emphasis on **trust** within ethical **guidance** as the basis for supporting joint decision making between professional and client.

The professional is expected to put the patient or client first in how they deploy their expertise. The adult client has the right to express their wishes and to expect that these will be respected in all but exceptional circumstances. Table 12.2 summarizes the main characteristics of these different approaches to ethics.

At first sight it would seem impossible to find ways of reconciling the differences. Each ethical approach is culturally embedded and has its own distinctive priorities. The conclusion of studies in the late 1990s was that it is impossible to produce a Europe-wide system of biomedical ethics that could usefully inform practice. To do so would involve disrespecting one or more cultures. However, the European Charter of Medical Ethics was agreed in 2011, which attempted a step in this direction (CEOM, 2011).

Whether it is possible for counsellors working with clients from very different cultural positions to work from a single ethical framework remains uncertain. The prevailing practice in the UK is to prioritize respect for client autonomy whilst maintaining a relationship of trust. A great deal depends on the interpretation of autonomy. Autonomy can be regarded as an ethic committed to endorsing individualism and therefore insensitive to clients whose identity is rooted in their extended family or wider community. The alternative approach is to view the self more flexibly so that the right to self-government can incorporate a range of different approaches to self-understanding. This approach to autonomy in professional ethics has a number of advantages as it is consistent with counsellors being attentive to, and working with, how a client understands their own situation. It may also solve a number of other issues. For example, an overemphasis on the self as a bounded individual free of ties and responsibilities to others does not represent the experience of many adults with dependent children or adults. There have been a number of analyses of autonomy from a feminist perspective that have convinced us that autonomy can encompass a range of self-understanding and that this is probably the best available way of deploying a professional ethic in the context of counselling. Making 'being **trustworthy**' the primary principle sets respect for autonomy within a relational context that can encompass considerable diversity in identities and relationships (Mackenzie and Stoljar, 2000).

As mental health and wellbeing are cultural constructs, practitioners not only need to adapt their practice to differences between understanding of self but also to what constitutes conditions that may benefit from counselling and other interventions. No single approach can accomplish this. The required approaches may be better understood within a larger framework, for example in the multicultural approaches to mental health to be found in Australia.

Ethics and Cultural Competence

For counsellors to work effectively across cultural differences, they need to ensure that they are adequately informed about the cultural background of their clients and that they are open psychologically to engaging with those differences. There are a number of ways of achieving this:

- *Attentive listening to the client and sensitively asking about potentially significant issues*: The strength of this approach lies in allowing the client to voice their understanding of their position within their culture and what they consider to be important. Relationships to one's own sub-cultures can be as varied as relationships between cultures. The limit to this approach is the potential for overburdening the client with educating the counsellor about cultural issues when they are wanting help with the issues that concern them.
- *Consulting the growing body of literature about cultural differences*: For example Laungani (2004); Moodley and West (2005); Lago (2008); Pedersen et al. (2008); and Ponterotto et al. (2009); Cousins (2019); Cameron (2020).
- *Seeking advice and supervision from someone who is well informed about the cultural characteristics and sensitivities*: This has the advantage of avoiding burdening the client with explaining their culture but care has to be taken over protecting client confidentiality, particularly if that client is from a community that is intensively networked.

- *Preparing ourselves to be psychologically open to cultural difference*: This is not usually a straightforward process. Engaging with other cultures often requires some appreciation of history and within that there will often have been conflicts and oppression. For counsellors with a European cultural background there may be some unpalatable truths to be faced about the way colonization was inflicted or achieved and the consequences of this. In her account of *Black Issues in the Therapeutic Process*, McKenzie-Mavinga (2009) observed how white counsellors might have to come to terms with 'recognition trauma' before they feel sufficiently comfortable to talk explicitly about racism and communicate freely with black people.

A commitment to non-discrimination is a necessary requirement in counselling ethics for working across differences between people but is not sufficient on its own. It is only the beginning of engaging with the other person, which requires a willingness to look beyond one's own personal and cultural assumptions in order to appreciate someone else's perspective on how to co-exist with people. In doing so we are ourselves personally and culturally transformed by our relationships with people who are different. It is not that we abandon our previous ethical points of reference but that these are understood in different ways (i.e. some strengths are appreciated more, new limitations are encountered, but above all new possibilities are opened up).

Pause for Reflection

What active steps do you take to reflect on your ethical position when working with clients from backgrounds very different to your own? What additional steps do you take to review with others (e.g. in supervision) that what you do is sufficient?

To accesss the online resources accompanying this chapter, please visit: https://study.sagepub.com/reevesandbond

Part III

The Counsellor and Others

13

Counsellors and the Responsibility to Others

Chapter Overview

This chapter provides an overview of different types of **responsibility** owed to the people affected by providing **counselling**, other than clients who are the focus of much of this book. Responsibility to oneself and to other counsellors, colleagues and members of the caring professions, as well as the wider community, are considered in turn.

Key words

self, colleagues, professionals, community

Responsibilities to the client are the primary concern of the counsellor but they are not the only responsibilities. There are other categories of **responsibility**. Any or all of these may impinge on how the responsibility to the client is implemented or occasionally may even take priority. Each of these is considered separately.

Responsibility to Self as a Counsellor

The ethical principle of **autonomy** is usually referred to in terms of **respect** for the client's capacity for self-determination. However, autonomy also applies to the counsellor; like clients, counsellors should only enter into a **counselling** relationship on a **voluntary** basis and as a result of having made a deliberate choice to do so. Counsellors also have an obligation to exercise care of themselves. Sometimes the ethical desirability of maintaining their own effectiveness, resilience and ability to help clients is understood solely as ensuring that a counsellor is competent to provide counselling and has the personal resources to do so. But behind this is an even more important principle. Counselling places considerable demands on counsellors, and there is always the risk of emotional burnout when working closely with the pain and **problems** of others. Counsellors have a responsibility to monitor their own responses and to protect their own wellbeing by avoiding excessive working and by making use of regular counselling **supervision**. Counselling supervision has a supportive role, but this is only one of the tasks addressed in supervision. Sometimes, it will be useful to supplement the support offered in supervision with personal counselling.

Tips for Self-care

The following points represent minimum **standards** of self-care. The optimum standard would include periodic reviews of whether providing counselling enriches a counsellor's quality of life. A great deal is said and written about the demands on counsellors, but if the only effect is personal depletion then why continue to do it? It is important to the mental health of the counsellor that there is also personal satisfaction in providing counselling.

Indemnity insurance

The importance of indemnity **insurance** from a client's point of view is considered in Chapter 5. There are also gains to the counsellor in terms of peace of mind. Even though the risks of having a claim made against a counsellor appear to be relatively small, should this arise the sums of money required even to obtain legal **advice** can be quite large. Adequate insurance helps to reduce the risk that the counsellor will incur unanticipated expenditure to compensate a client, and some insurance schemes also include free legal advice.

Personal safety

Fortunately, it is rare for counsellors to be physically or sexually attacked by clients, but it is not unknown; there have been very rare occasions where a counsellor has been killed by a client. It is important to keep in mind that some aspects of what might be considered 'good practice' might instead complicate a situation. For example, the counselling will usually take place away from other people in order to give the client **confidentiality** and **privacy**. This makes it harder for a counsellor to call for help. It is also not unusual for counselling rooms to be sited well away from busy areas to reduce extraneous noise. The same situation may arise if counsellors are working in their own home. This means that there may be no one close by to hear cries for help. The usual practice of taking clients who are not previously known to the counsellor, in order to maintain clarity about the nature of the relationship and professional **boundaries**, also creates an element of unpredictability and risk each time a counsellor takes on a new client.

Counsellors should organize their work in ways that will reduce the risk of assault on themselves. Counsellors who are vulnerable to assault have adopted two strategies, which can be implemented without compromising the **ethics** and **standards** of practice intended to protect the client:

- Taking referrals through someone else (e.g. GPs, **voluntary** organizations or colleagues) rather than seeing clients who walk in directly off the street or respond directly to advertisements.
- Making telephone contact whenever possible with clients before the first meeting; this provides a basic check on their physical location and gives the counsellor an opportunity to make a preliminary assessment.

Counsellors working with some client groups may not be able to implement any of these **safety** measures. For instance, counsellors who see clients with alcohol and drug **problems** may find that the potential benefits of a referral system for the counsellor's safety are outweighed by the deterrent effect this has on clients seeking counselling. Some clients do not have telephones or do not wish to have telephone calls from a counsellor because of the risk of someone they live with discovering they are receiving counselling. For example, a client seeking counselling about an extra-marital affair or a violent partner may have good reasons for not wanting a counsellor to make phone calls to their home.

However, all counsellors can take a number of basic precautions once a client arrives. These include:

- *Avoiding seeing new clients, or existing clients if there is any risk of assault, in an empty building*: It is better to have someone around who can be alerted by shouting or any unusual sounds. This is one of the advantages of counselling services that have receptionists or where counsellors share premises.
- *Providing the counselling rooms with telephones with outside lines*: If counsellors are seeing clients in premises with a switchboard operator telephone service, they may need a direct line to the public exchange when they see clients outside the usual working hours of the switchboard. Mobile phones only work as an alternative to land lines where there is a strong and reliable signal.
- *Installing an alarm or 'panic button'*: This may be particularly useful if there is a high level of risk to the counsellor.
- *Letting someone know in advance a specific time when the counsellor will contact them and giving them instructions about what to do if the counsellor fails to make contact*: It is much easier to handle a dangerous situation if all a counsellor has to do is contain it until help arrives, rather than having to take action to obtain help which may provoke the other person.

Likewise, as was discussed in Chapter 11, it is important for counsellors to take as much care for their personal safety when working online as when they work face to face. Careful use of social media sites, attention to the nature and type of personal information disclosed online (given that much can easily be traced, even with privacy settings in place) and the management of wider privacy settings when delivering counselling are non-negotiable considerations. These strategies may not prevent an assault, but they do increase the chance of obtaining assistance.

Care about Personal Safety?

A sense of personal safety is important if a counsellor is to feel secure enough to work creatively with clients. Sometimes counsellors will experience a sense of danger without any attack actually occurring. These feelings ought to be taken seriously and discussed in supervision. The sense of threat may arise from real danger, or a counsellor picking up a client's sense of threat to themself, or the re-stimulation of something from a counsellor's past. Whatever the cause, there is no ethical requirement for a counsellor to continue to see clients who evoke such feelings. A counsellor may refer a client to another counsellor if taking reasonable steps to promote safety is insufficient to reduce the sense of danger to an acceptable level.

Clients who harass counsellors outside the counselling relationship

It is rare for counsellors to be harassed by clients making nuisance phone calls, sending frequent unsolicited correspondence, or making unwelcome visits to a counsellor's home. However, 'stalking' and harassment of counsellors do happen from time to time, both face to face and online, based on information about a counsellor that the counsellor has posted on **social media** such as Facebook or Instagram. These are extremely distressing incidents for counsellors when they occur. The distress is compounded by the ethical constraints of confidentiality. Although ethical **guidance** seldom explicitly considers this kind of situation, a number of strategies are consistent with the ethics of counselling:

- Counselling supervision is important in providing emotional support for a counsellor as well as for reviewing potential courses of action.
- Medical and legal opinion may be sought about the client at an early stage. Providing the client's identity is not communicated, there is no breach of confidentiality. These consultations should take place with people who are unlikely to know the client.
- If the client is making public statements which are untrue and to the detriment of the counsellor, it may be appropriate to write to the client by recorded delivery or with a read receipt by email in the following terms: (a) any repetition of the statements by the client will be taken as an indication that the client regards the issue as no longer requiring confidentiality; (b) the counsellor will feel entitled to put their side of the story to those directly involved; and (c) the counsellor may contact solicitors, police, doctors and so on as appropriate.
- If the client persists after receiving a letter or email from the counsellor, then it is appropriate to consult solicitors to take action on the counsellor's behalf and sometimes it may be appropriate to contact the police.
- Events which happen outside the counselling relationship or after the counselling relationship has ended need not be treated as confidential.

Some situations have been resolved by the combination of a solicitor's letter and a refusal by the counsellor to enter into any further communication. All subsequent telephone calls and letters were ignored and eventually they stopped. However, the persistence of some clients can be remarkable and unfortunately just as distressing and disruptive to counsellors as any other form of persistent stalking or harassment. In such situations it may be necessary to seek legal advice about how best to stop the harassment.

These actions should be reserved for extreme situations. Counsellors do have to accept that from time to time clients will misrepresent what has happened within a counselling relationship. This most often happens when a counsellor is seeing one partner about difficulties in their relationship as a couple. Sometimes clients will attribute to the counsellor things that they are afraid to say for themselves (e.g. 'My counsellor says we should separate' or a college student might tell their parents that their counsellor says they should give up their course when this has not been the case). These situations are clearly potentially difficult, especially if the partner or parent approaches the counsellor directly. Nonetheless, the counsellor must maintain confidentiality by neither admitting nor denying what has happened in the counselling. (If a serious concern is being raised about the welfare of a young person, then it may be appropriate to follow **agency policy** where this exists, for example by making a referral to children's services.) Such incidents are on quite a different scale, however, from a situation where a client is seeking out a counsellor's colleagues or friends, or is persistently phoning late at night, or sending letters in disguised handwriting or emails from unnamed or disguised addresses to ensure they are opened by the counsellor.

Pause for Reflection

How do you manage self-disclosure online and what steps have you taken to attend to your safety by adjusting privacy settings?

Responsibility to Other Counsellors

Undermining public confidence in counselling

Counselling is only possible in a trusting relationship. The public reputation of counselling can create circumstances in which it is easier or harder to establish such a relationship. In order to protect the collective reputation of counselling and the reputation of members of any counselling organization there is a shared interest in protecting the public reputation of counsellors. Most counselling organizations attempt to protect their reputation for supporting good practice by requiring members to report concerns of any misconduct by other members and will expel members for behaviour that brings counselling into disrepute. The seriousness of what has occurred is also relevant in deciding whether public confidence in counselling has been undermined and brought into disrepute. Arguably, a fairly robust view has to be taken: for instance, two counsellors engaged in a heated public debate would not fall into this category unless either party became personally abusive and defamed the other or violence resulted.

A new area of concern, however, that has emerged over recent years, is how counsellors act on social media. Such platforms can provide an excellent space for debate, disagreement and challenge. Indeed, it might be argued that the profiling of discrimination or harm on social media has done much to bring such issues into public awareness. However, heated debate can quickly spill into personal abuse or threatening behaviour. Equally, counsellors sometimes draw on their client experiences to illustrate points they make online, without giving the same due care and attention to confidentiality that they might if using other media, such as in a publication. There continues to be much misunderstanding by some about the legality of posts on social media, which are contextualized by the same libel laws as any other public declaration. It is an area where counsellors are urged to proceed with great care and caution, and professional associations are slowly developing processes and guidance to attend to such situations.

Can a counsellor bring counselling into disrepute by activities unrelated to counselling? For example, if someone who works as a voluntary counsellor in their own time is convicted of fraud at their place of work, would this amount to bringing counselling into disrepute? Most professional organizations require members to notify them of criminal convictions and will consider whether the conviction is compatible with continued membership of that organization. **Insurance** companies will also ask for information about any convictions and this may impact on the cover given or the cost of the premium. Recent criminal convictions, especially those involving deception or violence, can bring the profession into disrepute.

Responsibility to Colleagues and Members of the Caring Professions

Accountability to others

Counsellors working on their own in private practice are largely free of the need to be accountable to anyone other than their clients and can discuss any difficulties with a counselling supervisor. However, counselling is increasingly provided within organizations involving more complex patterns of **accountability** to managers, committees and others.

There have been situations in which it has seemed that counsellors have wanted to use confidentiality as a shield to protect them from appropriate accountability to colleagues. For example, confidentiality has been used as an excuse for avoiding **disclosure** that a large number of clients are missing their appointments, or to avoid accountability for resources being used. This is an abuse of confidentiality. However, the methods used in being accountable should be consistent with the ethics and standards of practice of counselling. What this means in practice is considered in detail in Chapter 14.

A counsellor's responsibility to increase colleagues' understanding

Counsellors report that the voluntary nature of counselling and the need for confidentiality are the two aspects of counselling that most frequently give rise to misunderstandings. It takes positive action by counsellors working in organizations to develop appropriate expectations of counselling. Sometimes clients and colleagues will have inappropriate expectations of a counsellor's role. For example, a tutor may refer a young person with an eating disorder for counselling and assume that the counsellor will also monitor the client's weight and general health. These are inappropriate expectations. Weighing the client and any health checks would need to be carried out by someone with medical or nursing qualifications.

Responsibility to the Wider Community

The ethical focus is usually on the client–counsellor relationship rather than on social units like the family, except for counsellors working primarily with families or the wider community. However, there will be some situations where a counsellor is faced with **dilemmas** concerning responsibilities to the wider community.

One recurrent issue is what to do if a client talks about committing or having committed serious crimes.

Pause for Reflection

Sheila talks about her distress at being involved in a robbery in which someone was injured. She also mentions plans for another robbery in one week's time. What should the counsellor do?

Does the counsellor have a duty to report the crime that has been committed? There is no general duty in criminal **law** to report to the police or anyone else that a client has committed a crime. (Statutory exceptions are considered in Chapter 10.) There is also no general duty to answer police questions about a client. A polite but clear refusal to answer is all that is required. However, to give false or misleading answers can amount to the offence of wasting police time or obstructing a police officer in the execution of their duty.

Does the counsellor have a duty to prevent crime? There is no general duty under criminal law to prevent someone committing a crime outside the counselling room, with the exception of statutory requirements to notify the authorities of information held about particular offences, like terrorism (see Chapter 10). If the crime is being committed within the counselling session, then the legal position is rather different. A counsellor who failed to prevent or take reasonable steps to prevent an offence in the counsellor's presence may have committed the offences of aiding and abetting, or 'counselling' (in the criminal law sense of being an accomplice to a crime). This would arise only if the counsellor's inactivity amounted to positive encouragement. A counsellor is most likely to be charged with these offences when a client assaults another, uses illegal drugs, or attempts **suicide** in the presence of the counsellor.

There is a right, but not a duty, to use such force as is reasonable in the circumstances to prevent crime. Some crimes are not serious enough to justify the use of force. Illegal drug use may come into this category. The use of more force than is reasonable is in itself a crime. Therefore, the use of physical restraint to stop someone hitting another person is usually reasonable, but the use of a weapon would not be. Because suicide is no longer a crime, there is no general right to use reasonable force to prevent suicide attempts or suicide (see Chapter 7 for a further discussion of this issue).

Could the counsellor inadvertently incur liability for a client's acts? The answer is 'yes'. The following example illustrates how a counsellor could commit the criminal offence of incitement.

Suppose the counsellor honestly but mistakenly believes that it is not illegal for his 15-year-old male client to engage in sexual intercourse in private with another consenting male of the same age. Consequently, the counsellor encourages and supports his client in sexual experimentation of this nature as part of his 'homework' assignment.

It is not necessary for the counsellor to know that the activity is an offence for the counsellor to be guilty of incitement. (The current age of consent for homosexual acts between men is 16 years old in the UK and 17 in Eire.) The counsellor may not want his client to break the law. It is sufficient that the law has been broken for the offence to have been committed, although the counsellor's mistake about the law and lack of deliberate intention to incite an offence would be taken into account in sentencing. It is therefore wise to be cautious when setting the client tasks between sessions, a technique frequently used in behavioural methods of counselling. Dryden and Neenan (2004) caution that 'Whatever behavioural assignment you negotiate with your client, ensure it is both legal and ethical.'

A counsellor can also incur civil liability for inciting or encouraging a client to break a **contract** with a third party. For example, a counsellor encourages a client to change jobs without giving the contracted amount of notice to the first employer or to stop supplying goods that the client has contracted to provide. If the client carries out the act, which has been encouraged, the counsellor may become jointly liable for any resulting loss to a third party. It is also possible that the counsellor could be jointly liable for a client's breach of confidence that has been incited by the counsellor.

While there is not a great deal of evidence of the likelihood of this, it is a theoretical possibility that a counsellor could be prosecuted or sued for incitement of a client's wrongdoing. At a workshop, Kenneth Cohen (1992) cautioned counsellors to be careful when using empathic responses with a client who is intending to commit an unlawful act. The counsellor has to choose between being empathic, which the client often interprets as encouragement, and the possibility, albeit a remote one, of incurring legal liabilities as a consequence of the client's subsequent acts or withholding empathy.

Ethical dilemmas that do not necessarily involve the law can also arise, as in the following example.

Edward uses counselling to ease his guilt about deceiving his partner about his frequent sexual relationships with other people. Sheila, the counsellor, feels increasingly concerned on behalf of his partner.

The ethics of respecting the client's autonomy and confidentiality would prevent the counsellor from communicating her concern to the partner directly. But what if Edward has a life-threatening **illness** with which he could infect his partner? This makes the ethical dilemma much more acute. This has arisen in HIV/AIDS counselling. The general practice has been to respect the client's control over confidential information but to work in ways which make it easier for him to tell his partner, including offering to be present when he tells them. Occasionally, counsellors have told partners with the client's consent or at the client's request. Alternatively, clients have, often of their own volition, chosen to abstain from doing anything that would put their partner at risk of infection until they feel able to tell them about their health problem. Some clients prefer to abstain from sex or other activities that would put their partner at risk for the rest of their lives, rather than tell that partner. But what if the client deliberately and recklessly continues to put a partner at risk of infection? This would appear to be a situation in which, after consultation with the client and other experienced counsellors, the counsellor might decide it is defensible to break confidentiality to warn the partner (see Chapter 10). There has been an increasing tendency to prosecute people who knowingly put others at risk of HIV infection. The seriousness of the situation for everyone involved means that the counsellor needs to be sure that there is no possible alternative course of action.

Conclusion

The management of conflicting responsibilities is particularly challenging for a counsellor. Whenever possible, it is better to anticipate what these might be and find ways of avoiding them. If such a conflict cannot be avoided, then it is important that the client knows of this so that either the contract between the counsellor and client can take these into account or the client can seek counselling elsewhere. These situations are much easier to handle prospectively than retrospectively. One of the best ways to be forewarned of potential conflicts of responsibility is to discuss situations with an experienced counsellor working in a similar situation. This is one of the key functions of counselling supervision.

Pause for Reflection

How regularly do you discuss in supervision the responsibilities to others you hold in virtue of your counselling role? If you work as a counsellor in different contexts, do these responsibilities differ?

To access the online resources accompanying this chapter, please visit: https://study.sagepub.com/reevesandbond

14

Counselling Supervision

Chapter Overview

Counselling supervision, used in the education and training of counsellors and in the UK and some other countries, is an ongoing requirement throughout the working life of a counsellor. This chapter considers the ethical basis of supervision and the different tasks and modes involved. It concludes with three examples of **issues** that might well be presented in supervision and as examples of how supervision addresses ethical and therapeutic issues.

Key words

counselling supervision, normative, formative, restorative, perspective

Supervision has a long history that goes back to the origins of the talking therapies. Both the early Freudians and Jungians appear to have developed forms of supervision to support psychoanalysts with the dynamic aspects of their work, particularly the unconscious elements at work between therapist and client. It is as true now as it was in the origins of psychoanalysis that it is considered helpful to have someone familiar with the psychology of relationships and human interactions to assist therapists in understanding their work with clients. Many counsellors would not use psychoanalysis directly and prefer other approaches to their work but recognize the value of an ongoing working relationship with someone to discuss their **counselling**. Most professional bodies for counselling require that counsellors receive regular and ongoing supervision (BPS, 2018; IACP, 2018; BACP, 2018a; UKCP, 2019). Ongoing supervision has been widely accepted as an essential protection of professional and especially **ethical standards** within the UK. However, there are critics of supervision requirements, especially for experienced counsellors. The discussion will begin by exploring what supervision is and how it supports ethical practice throughout the early stages of a counsellor's career, before turning to the more problematic aspects of supervision.

What is Counselling Supervision?

Most definitions of supervision have several elements in common, even if the precise words are different. Counselling supervision is characterized by:

- being primarily directed to enhancing the service to clients, although operating indirectly through the counsellor;
- a degree of formality, with explicit agreements about working arrangements for the supervision, including the regularity of sessions, the allocation of **responsibility** for the client work, **confidentiality** and any payments;
- protecting ethical **standards** both individually and collectively for counsellors;
- protecting and enhancing standards of practice;
- operating with some independence from direct line management or **accountability** to professional bodies in order to provide sufficient **privacy** for the counsellor to work with the personal **issues** involved in the work;
- supporting the counsellor's wellbeing and capability to undertake an emotionally challenging role.

All of these elements are brought together with varying degrees of emphasis in the following definitions:

> Supervision is essential to how practitioners sustain good practice throughout their working life. Supervision provides practitioners with regular and ongoing opportunities to reflect in depth about all aspects of their practice in order to work as effectively, safely and ethically as possible. Supervision also sustains the personal resourcefulness required to undertake the work. (BACP, 2018a: 22)
>
> The objectives of consultation/supervision are:
>
> - to provide practitioners with consultation on their work with clients;
> - to enhance the quality and competence of practice offered to all clients;

- to offer psychologists intellectual challenge enabling reflection, transformational learning and psychological support to maximise their responsibility for appropriate self-care; and
- to contribute to the CPD of both psychologist and supervisor by developing competence in the use and practise of supervision. (BPS, 2017: 13)

Essentially, therefore, the purpose of professional supervision is for counsellors to reflect on and develop effective and ethical practice within a secure and ongoing relationship. This may include monitoring work with clients. Supervision includes personal support, working at relational depth, mentoring, professional development, and provides opportunities to reflect on relationships between people, theories, practices, work contexts and cultural perspectives.

International Variations in Approaches to Counselling Supervision

Various countries have developed their counselling supervision in distinctive ways. In the USA, counselling supervision is primarily directed at developing trainee counsellors and is replaced by a system of consultation with experienced colleagues when supervision is no longer required after qualification. It is very closely associated with counsellor education and is adapted as counsellors move from the dependence and naïveté of a novice towards independent practice through a developmental approach to supervision (Stoltenberg and Delworth, 1987). The British approach to supervision is different: it is envisaged that supervision will continue throughout the working life of a counsellor, both as form of professional **accountability** in the interests of clients and for the professional and personal development of the counsellor.

Hawkins and Shohet (2012) identify seven modes of supervision that capture different elements of the triangular relationship between client, counsellor and supervisor:

1. A focus on the client and what and how they present.
2. An exploration of the strategies and interventions used by the supervisee.
3. A focus on the relationship between client and supervisee.
4. A focus on the supervisee.
5. A focus on the supervisory relationship.
6. The supervisor focusing on their own process.
7. A focus on the wider contexts in which the work happens (and what these mean to the client, supervisee and supervisor).

This emphasis on process is also evident in the other widely used model of supervision in the UK, the cyclical model of Page and Wosket (2014), which describes the reflective space offered by supervision in terms of a cycle made up of five stages:

1. Contracting about ground rules and expectations of each other.
2. Agreeing a focus.
3. Making a space for reflection.
4. Building the link between supervision and work with the client.
5. Review and evaluation.

They envisage that the counsellor and supervisor will keep revisiting these stages in a cyclical manner, thereby strengthening both the supervision and the counselling.

In both the UK and the USA, it is assumed that the supervisor will be from within the profession of counselling and suitably trained in both counselling and supervision. European traditions appear less restrictive and are more open to supervision across professions. Supervisors are not restricted to work within their own professions and may apply their skills and knowledge of supervision across a wide range of different types of workers with people (Carroll and Holloway, 1999; Carroll, 2014).

International comparisons between approaches to supervision reveal another distinction, explored later in this chapter. The movement of people between countries and the growth of working online means that counsellors increasingly face the challenges and opportunities of working with clients from outside their own cultural background. Counsellors in New Zealand appear particularly aware of this challenge because of the sensitivities and tensions between the Maori as the long-standing inhabitants of those islands and the westerners or *pakeha* in a constitutional framework of biculturalism. In reality, New Zealand is becoming rapidly multicultural as people from other cultures in Asia and the Pacific settle alongside Maori and Europeans. The implications of providing counselling across **cultural differences** are also particularly evident in North America, as discussed in Chapter 12. The ethical challenges of cultural difference are taken sufficiently seriously for supervision to be seen as having a major role to play in developing culturally appropriate services and supporting counsellors in understanding the unfamiliar. In some cases, a supervisor will be selected because of their specific cultural knowledge and background and will fulfil all the functions of supervision. Alternatively, the cultural supervision may be provided to supplement the usual counselling supervision from within a specific cultural **identity**. This use of supervision to address cultural differences is not wholly absent from British approaches to counselling, but is much less prominent in published **ethics** by professional bodies in the UK in comparison to New Zealand and North America.

The Tasks of Counselling Supervision

Counselling supervision is intended to make a major contribution to the ethical integrity of the work with clients; this is only one of several functions. The pioneers of supervision training in the UK (Inskipp, 1986; Proctor, 1988; Inskipp and Proctor, 1994, 1995) developed supervision to address three core tasks:

1. *Normative:* establishing and protecting professional ethics and standards of practice.
2. *Formative:* enhancing the aptitude, knowledge and skills of the counsellor (a form of continuing professional development focusing on work with current clients).
3. *Restorative:* supporting the counsellor with the personal effects of working closely with people who may be experiencing considerable distress or difficulty. The preventative function is to reduce the counsellor's risk of burnout or secondary traumatization. Providing a degree of personal support is also intended to prevent the counsellor from becoming so self-protective against emotional pain that they are unable to form empathic or effective relationships with clients. It also works positively to affirm the value of this type of intervention to keep the counsellor motivated and energized for providing counselling.

As a result of researching counsellors working in multidisciplinary teams, Bond (1991) added:

4. *Perspective:* an opportunity to see counselling in the wider professional context of other services and social systems and to reflect on how to maximize any benefits to the client. (See Table 14.1.)

TABLE 14.1 *The tasks of counselling supervision: template for dividing tasks*

		Undertaken by	
Task	**Description**	**Line manager**	**Counselling supervisor/ consultative support**
Formative	Skill development; reflection on experience; new understanding; new knowledge about counselling process, client group, specific issues raised by client		
Normative	Counselling: standards; ethics and practice; agency: standards; ethics and practice; monitoring the quality of counselling; consideration of feedback from client		

(Continued)

TABLE 14.1 *(Continued)*

		Undertaken by	
Task	**Description**	**Line manager**	**Counselling supervisor/ consultative support**
Restorative	Dealing with personal issues and stress arising from counselling; validating achievements		
Perspective	Overview of total counselling work; relationship between counselling and other methods of clients obtaining help; relationships with counsellors and members of other professions		

Counselling supervision is about much more than ethics. It is a mixture of ethics and 'practices', in which the overall impact comes from the supervisor modelling good practice that influences the counsellor positively (Houston, 1995). Modelling is a very powerful influence that operates both consciously and subliminally and can enhance good practice. Unfortunately, poor modelling in supervision can also undermine good practice and encourage poor practice.

Pause for Reflection

Consider what you look for in supervision. If you are a trainee, how does that inform and shape your learning on your programme? If you are a qualified counsellor, have your supervisory needs changed as you have built up more experience?

Ethical Dimensions of Counselling Supervision

Boundaries between professional and personal relationships

Maintaining **boundaries** between the supervisor and supervisee has long been considered as important as between counsellor and client; there are probably two main reasons for this. The first is sustaining a model that supports the management of boundaried relationships between counsellors and clients. Behavioural modelling is a powerful way of reinforcing or undermining learning for other relationships. The second reason is that a substantial part of the justification for the supervisory relationship in counselling is one of professional accountability, and such accountability can be clouded by possible confusion with line management issues, divided loyalties, friendship and close personal relationships. Some supervisory relationships can start out with clear relational boundaries but then become closer over time.

Sheila has supervised Bob's counselling for over three years. They have developed mutual respect for each other and have successfully managed encountering each other in a local counselling association at training events and have been able to keep a boundary between being sociable at these local events and working in greater depth in supervision. They both enjoy walking and without any knowledge of each other's arrangements have booked on the same ramblers' weekend, staying in the same hostel. When they discover this, they start to question where the boundaries lie in the relationship for supervisor and supervisee.

This would be an appropriate point to review how far it is possible to maintain the boundaries in a supervisory relationship in ways that are professionally credible to others regardless of how scrupulous the two people concerned are. Some people are better than others at maintaining boundaries. Even if there is no intention for the friendship to develop further, it may be worth the supervisee considering finding a new supervisor and reflecting on how future social contacts with the former supervisor will be maintained. Where this is not practical, perhaps due to a shortage of suitable supervisors, it may be wise to adopt deliberate strategies to ensure clearer boundaries between the professional and personal roles. Some approaches to counselling are more open to combining friendship with a professional role in a considered way in comparison to others. All these factors need to be taken into account. This is the sort of situation that requires careful consideration by the people involved and may be relatively unproblematic on some occasions and possibly quite problematic in others.

Who is responsible for the counselling delivered to the client?

The general principle is that there is a chain of responsibility from the client to the counsellor and then from the counsellor to the supervisor. Supervisors do not normally assume a direct responsibility to clients. They work to enhance the counselling work and the benefits for clients through supervisees. The following example raises the issue of whether this ought to be the approach to responsibility for work with clients.

Hubert is a trainee counsellor who is developing good basic skills but is not yet confident in moving from what clients say to selecting the most appropriate counselling actions to help them. He presents a case in supervision where he considers that the client and he are going around in repetitive circles and the client's circumstances are deteriorating. As Hubert's supervisor, Pam is sufficiently concerned for the client that she is questioning her responsibilities to the client and the trainee counsellor.

A great deal will depend on the modality of the practitioner and expectations of therapy, the degree of vulnerability of the client and the severity of their **problems**. If we suppose that the client's deterioration is putting them seriously at risk of **self-harm**, and Hubert as the counsellor seems both overwhelmed and helpless, in such circumstances a supervisor may feel that the normative and protective functions of supervision ought to carry greater weight than the formative support of the supervisee. An experienced supervisor will explore a range of possible options before taking the exceptional act (see below) of intervening directly by offering to see the client personally. It may be that Hubert can be supported in seeking additional support or making a referral to a more experienced or suitable counsellor. Such an approach would have the advantage of supporting Hubert to recognize the boundaries to his **competence** and how to manage such situations in future. However, this will only work if there is a real prospect of meeting the client's needs at the same time as developing the trainee counsellor.

Similarly, there may be resources on Hubert's course that could be brought into play or, alternatively, from within the counselling service where Hubert is seeing the client. In an extreme situation, the priority ought to be the protection of the client's best interests. In the absence of any other possibility, it may be justified for the supervisor to arrange a meeting with the client through Hubert in order to undertake an assessment to ensure that the client's needs can be met by a suitable referral or through a better-supported Hubert. One of the difficulties thereafter is that the supervisor takes on potentially conflicting responsibilities to the client and the trainee. In order to prevent such an eventuality, most supervisors of trainees will ensure that the counselling agency and the training course take primary responsibilities in backing up the work of the trainee where a client is considered to be at risk. The arrangements for communicating any concerns would have formed part of the working agreement between the supervisor and supervisee and ought to be consistent with the agreement between the client and the trainee. In the example, the concerns were raised through the trainee counsellor. What if these had been raised by the client directly? A concerned client ought to be directed to raise their concerns with the counselling agency in the first instance rather than with the training course or the supervisor.

Some clients are faced with deteriorating circumstances that may be beyond any reasonable expectations of a trainee counsellor or even beyond the range of a competent experienced counsellor. A sound assessment procedure before allocation minimizes such occurrences but cannot wholly eliminate them. Life happens. In fairness to both clients and trainees, it is important to have plans in place for such eventualities.

Supporting supervisees taking on new approaches to providing counselling

It is increasingly common for clients to want to communicate with their counsellors online. For some clients this may be simply arranging appointments by email or text, but what if this is wanting to receive counselling online rather than face to face? This has become a particular issue as a result of the COVID-19 pandemic, causing in-person counselling services to be closed and the majority of counsellors, many for the first time, being forced to work online. Likewise, their supervisors were faced with the challenge of making an overnight and apparently seamless switch to delivering supervision online. This online shift, for some a positive decision they had made pre-pandemic, became a new normal. However, early evidence suggests that many counsellors, having experienced the advantages of working online, intend to retain that approach either fully or, at least, in a blended way; this may be true for supervisors also. This shift naturally raised particular issues for trainees working towards their practice hours in order to qualify: training programmes were challenged to think about introducing modules about working online to equip their trainees for this new environment, and indeed to deliver training and teaching online too.

Jane is a competent face-to-face counsellor and very capable with new technology in other areas of her life. She has a young family and is looking for ways to be able to work from home in dedicated blocks of time around her support with childcare. She greatly values her supervisor's insights and has found that her current supervision has greatly enhanced her work with her face-to-face clients. She is not in a position to take time out for substantial further training but would like to develop an online counselling service for mothers with young children. She raises this possibility with her supervisor, who is doubtful about the potential of online counselling.

This is a situation which challenges both counsellor and supervisor alike. The ethical issue for both is offering services within their competence. How far is it feasible or ethically acceptable to offer services in a new format without any training? Training does not have to be within a classroom at some inconvenient distance from the home. It can be **online** and in these circumstances may be the most appropriate way forward. As the counsellor has demonstrated good basic competence in face-to-face counselling and an openness to learning, it may be that other forms of informal learning will also be highly appropriate, such as reading around the growing literature (Jones and Stokes, 2009; Evans, 2009; Stokes, 2018; Weinberg and Rolnick, 2019) and discussing this as a part of supervision. The supervisor is also faced with questioning his conservatism or willingness to innovate and what the boundaries are for his competence. Is it possible to supervise competently in areas where the supervisor has no previous experience? There may also be some gendered prejudices about the opportunities available to women with families. If the supervisor is at the edge of his comfort zone and competence, it may be more appropriate for the supervisee to seek a new supervisor for this component or all her supervision. One possibility would be online supervision.

However the supervision is carried forward, there will be a need to consider appropriate online methods for offering counselling, developing the relevant skills (e.g. how to communicate core counselling skills in a different means of communication rather than in person), developing contracts appropriate to the medium of working, ensuring confidentiality and **security**, meeting data protection requirements, and the other issues that will inevitably arise. Whether or not it is in a supervisory role or some other form of support, there is strong case here for the counsellor joining a network of like-minded counsellors to accelerate her familiarity with the issues and how they can be resolved.

Pause for Reflection

If you were a trainee or qualified counsellor what challenges did you encounter in your work as a result of restrictions imposed because of the COVID-19 pandemic: both in terms of delivering counselling, but also how or whether lockdown shaped the nature of presenting problems? How did you use supervision to navigate these challenges?

Working with clients across cultural differences

The challenges of working across cultural differences are often rooted in the particular cultures of the people involved and our willingness to see beyond what is familiar.

In social contact, this is a two-way responsibility. The emphasis on clients' needs in counselling places a greater responsibility on counsellors to be culturally informed and to communicate in culturally appropriate ways. Clients ought to be freed from the burden of educating their counsellors in cultural issues in much the same way as a client would not be expected to educate a counsellor in the basics of depression or the techniques of a particular approach to counselling. This may be easier said than done, however. The experience of distress is socially constructed and often culturally specific so physical, emotional or social problems will be understood and experienced very differently in different cultures, if they are recognized at all. Counselling requires counsellors to become adept at listening beyond their own personal experience, but it takes on new dimensions when listening across cultural differences.

Bill presents a case in supervision about his work with Aneeta, a young Asian woman who is increasingly concerned that her family want her to marry a cousin as part of their plans for strengthening family cohesion and the family business. She is the first generation of her family to be educated in the UK and feels caught between her loyalty to her parents and her respect for their wishes against her desire to have a more independent life, like many of her friends. Bill is familiar with counselling about tensions between young adult children and their parents, but is unsure of the significance of cultural differences and whether there are culturally appropriate ways of responding. His gender does not appear to be an issue for this client, but he is aware that it would be an issue for her parents, who seem to want to protect their daughter from male company. Rachel, his supervisor, like Bill, has limited experience of this particular community originating from a northern region in India. They discuss how best to acquire this knowledge and how far it is appropriate to rely on this client to educate her counsellor.

Cultural perspectives can be shaped by the cultural context in which the counsellor lives. This example is fairly typical for most parts of the UK, with the counsellor being part of an indigenous majority recognizing a responsibility to be culturally better informed. There is growing literature on both sides of the Atlantic for all professions working across cultures and some very useful books specifically for counsellors (Lago, 2008; Cousins, 2019; Cameron, 2020). In this case, it may be appropriate to seek some supplementary **mentoring** or supervision from someone familiar with the **culture**. However, caution may be required. If the cultural group is small and well known to each other, it may be impossible to seek mentoring from within this group without risking client anonymity. In most cases, it would be desirable for a client to be consulted about what issues it would be helpful for the counsellor to understand better and whether any of the possible ways of acquiring the knowledge are acceptable to the client. Great care and sensitivity may also be required when working with refugees as the client's concern to protect family members in another country may be a much greater priority than receiving help through counselling. Services that routinely work across cultures may wish to build cultural awareness into their training and staff development processes.

The strong association between culture, **identity** and ethics is so intermeshed that ethical assumptions behind most approaches to counselling may not translate well between cultures (Bond, 2007). Being **trustworthy** may be a better starting point than prioritizing **respect** for **autonomy**. This is particularly so where someone's identity is strongly associated with a family group or clan rather than they as an individual. (For further discussion, see Chapters 12 and 16, and Bond, 2007.)

How Ethical Is the Current Requirement for Regular and Ongoing Supervision?

This might seem to be an absurd question when counselling supervision has been adopted internationally as one of the ethical safeguards of counselling. However, there are some legitimate questions to be posed from an ethical perspective.

1. Are the resources and time consumed by supervision justified or could these resources be better invested to the benefit of clients and counselling?

This is a question about **justice** and fairness in the distribution of finite and often limited resources. Counselling supervision is resource-intensive because it requires the attention of two professionals simultaneously, the supervisor and counsellor, in circumstances where one or both may need to be paid. There is also a substantial opportunity cost as both could be providing frontline counselling services in the time devoted to supervision. It requires some substantial and well-evidenced benefits in order to justify such a recurrent and long-term use of resources as a strict obligation.

2. What is the evidence for the benefits of counselling supervision?

Frankly, the evidence is not as convincing as one might hope. Perhaps this should not be surprising because it is only relatively recently that the evidence for the effectiveness of counselling based on credible **research** has accumulated (Wheeler and Richards, 2007; Cooper, 2008). Researching the impact of counselling supervision is more complex. It is extremely difficult to establish a causal relationship between what happens in supervision and the benefits to the client. We experience this subjectively, but it is hard to demonstrate to scientific standards.

Nevertheless, anecdotal evidence and personal experience are generally positive about the effects of supervision on the counsellor and, through the counsellor, on the client. A systematic review of the available research evidence concluded that although the quality of the research evidence is variable, supervision is consistently demonstrated to have positive effects on the supervisee. The research evidence of beneficial effects on counsellors is strongest for trainee counsellors and less certain for experienced or qualified counsellors. Little is reliably known about the impact on client outcome (Wheeler and Richards, 2007).

3. Does supervision involve some inherent violation of being respectful of clients' rights to privacy and confidentiality that are increasingly recognized in the moral and legal frameworks of contemporary society?

Unless managed ethically, it is possible for supervision to violate client **rights** and particularly client **privacy**. Counsellors do not know every aspect of their clients' lives; in particular, they are unlikely to know to whom a client is an identifiable person. Even if the name of a client is not disclosed in supervision, it is possible that a supervisor may identify them from incidental details. Only the client is well placed to make these judgments and decide the level of risk that is acceptable. On balance, good practice suggests that a client ought to be informed about the counsellor's supervision arrangements, including the name of their supervisor. This enables the client to consider whether they are willing to be discussed on an anonymized basis, first name only or as an identifiable person and to give consent. It also gives a client the ability to consider whether they might know the supervisor in some way, and to evaluate for themselves any possible difficulty or conflict of interest if they should be identified or become identifiable within supervision. This is particularly important in situations where the counsellor, supervisor and client all live or work within a small community.

4. What is the impact of compulsory, ongoing supervision on the ethical performance of counselling?

As counselling takes place mostly in private under conditions of confidentiality, widening the visibility of the work to the constructive scrutiny of a supervisor is probably a useful ethical safeguard. It is probably most effective as a safeguard against unethical practice by counsellors who are well intentioned but drift into poor practice through ignorance or mistake. Where supervision is provided to high standards, it provides a positive influence towards higher standards and the enhancement of ethical and professional standards.

Developments in Supervision

While supervision in its current form has been established for many years, practice developments around supervision continue, in terms of forms of delivery (face to face, online, chat-based, avatar) as well as the broader purpose and function. This is particularly true in the *application* of counselling supervision to other roles and situations beyond the traditional counselling relationship. Other professional groups, such as teachers, mental health workers, social workers and nurses, are beginning to develop greater supervisory awareness that goes beyond their more traditional case-management style. The literature on compassion fatigue and vicarious trauma (Brown, 2017) sheds further light on the impact of vocational work beyond that encountered in the therapy world. The following example illustrates one application of the principles of a supervisory process beyond a traditional supervisory relationship.

University managers have become increasingly aware of the impact on their disability support staff of direct work with students presenting with physical and emotional health needs. These demands are often high and not uncommonly include risk of self-harm and suicide potential. Disability support workers have not received specific training in this area, are not counsellors or mental health workers, but provide a frontline response, often in crisis situations. Having discussed concerns with the University Counselling Service, they agree to establish a Reflective Practice Group (RPG). This RPG will meet every six weeks and be attended by all 12 disability support workers. It will be facilitated by an experienced and qualified counsellor/supervisor from the Counselling Service. They will draw on the formative, normative, restorative and perspective principles outlined above, but will not be offering the depth of supervisory process that might be experienced in a traditional counselling frame. While this will be a culturally new experience, the disability support workers find huge benefit in being able to talk, confidentially, about the impact of their work, to receive support, guidance and to ensure they are working safely.

An RPG, as an example of the principles of supervision used in an applied way, illustrates how the learning gleaned over many years of supervisory practice and theoretical development can be used to support and enhance work in other contexts.

Finally, some case examples to illustrate some of the possible benefits of counselling supervision perhaps shed some light on why supervision remains an ethical requirement for many counsellors, even though the research evidence remains patchy.

Example 1

The counsellor is working with a client, David (19 years old), who is using counselling to look at the impact of an eating disorder on his relationships, particularly with his girlfriend. His eating disorder has not improved and is showing signs of deteriorating. His counsellor wishes to refer David for more specialized treatment than she feels able to offer. David refuses and insists on continuing to work with her.

Trust and reaching the limits of competence

David has a severe and continuing eating disorder that seems to be getting worse. Nonetheless he trusts his counsellor and does not want to be referred for more specialist help. How ought the counsellor to respond to his desire to continue work with her against her concern that he may need a different type of help?

This is a challenging situation for which counselling supervision provides an opportunity to the counsellor to think through the potentially conflicting issues. She is faced with a situation that requires her to think how best to respond to:

- reaching the limits of her competence;
- respecting her client's **trust** and autonomy;
- managing confidentiality;
- considering whether she has any duty to intervene in the best interests of her client.

It is often difficult to think through the issues carefully without an opportunity to discuss them with someone outside the counselling relationship. The first issue points towards making a change in how counselling is offered, and referral is the obvious but not the only solution. The second and third issues point to continuing to work with the client as referral and the **disclosure** of confidential material require his consent. The final issue is not applicable as this client is an adult, but nonetheless the counsellor feels a commitment to act in his best interests.

A skilled supervisor will help the counsellor think through how to balance these conflicting demands and their ethical and therapeutic implications. The counsellor is faced with a choice between:

- refusing to continue to work with the client and offering referral as the only alternative to no counselling;
- continuing to see the client with additional expert support and supervision, which would require the client's consent;
- continue to see the client but rapidly train to acquire the relevant knowledge and skills;
- continue to work with the client without any change.

Pause for Reflection

What do you consider to be the more ethically appropriate outcomes? Which would you choose in a similar situation?

Example 2

The counsellor, Emily, is feeling stuck and distressed on behalf of a student client who is likely to fail his course because he is refusing to accept help for his dyslexia. Supervision is an ideal place to discuss such cases.

Supervision supporting ethical practice

This supervisee is talking about a client, Chris, who causes her concern because he won't accept the help on offer to him. She feels stuck and frustrated. What are the ethical and therapeutic issues that supervision could helpfully address? How can the quality of counselling being offered be improved by supervision?

Feeling stuck with a client and not knowing what to do for the best can have many causes, including:

- not knowing what to do because of reaching the limits of professional knowledge or skills;
- overlooking something that is significant in what the client is presenting, consciously or unconsciously;
- an unacknowledged obstacle in the counsellor's mind, often referred to as projection or countertransference in some approaches to counselling;
- a contextual issue that seems to limit the options or block a way forward.

A skilled supervisor can help the counsellor/supervisee identify the causes of feeling stuck and turn an obstacle into a positive insight that helps to move the counselling forward.

Example 3

The supervisee, Emily, has noticed a change in how she is working with clients. The cause is not immediately obvious to her. She is concerned that building relationships with new clients, something she normally does well, no longer seems to be happening.

Counsellor self-care

We all counsel against the backdrop of our lives. Emily has noticed having some unfamiliar reactions and difficulties with her clients. What does the supervisor do to help her consider these more deeply and what are the benefits or potential risks to her clients?

Relationship building is an essential part of counselling in all approaches. Emily is right to be concerned and to consider this to be a sufficiently serious issue to present in supervision.

There can be many causes of failing to form relationships with clients:

- Some clients may mistrust the counsellor or be prejudiced against the counsellor's characteristics.
- Social **diversity** can create bigger gaps between people than either the client or counsellor feels able or willing to jump.
- Counsellors may struggle to find the emotional energy or resourcefulness to build a relationship.
- There may be deep-seated psychological barriers to forming relationships.
- Counsellors will encounter all these and possibly other obstacles to relationship building in their work. Supervision can help to examine what is happening in any particular relationship.

Pause for Reflection

In this example, the supervisee has lost the capability to form relationships that she has demonstrated in the past. Which of the listed explanations seems most likely to apply? How would you expect her supervisor to help her?

Self-care is an ethical issue in counselling. Sometimes supervision is sufficient to return us to our normal functioning. However, the supportive function of supervision is constrained by other tasks. In some cases, counselling for the counsellor may be required.

To access the online resources accompanying this chapter, please visit: https://study.sagepub.com/reevesandbond

15

Record-keeping

Chapter Overview

Record-keeping is widely accepted as an ethical requirement for good practice. This chapter examines the ethical basis for keeping or not keeping **records**, and the significance of records being kept securely. Ethical **issues** around clients' access to their records and their use in courts are considered. The chapter concludes with how records ought to be written.

Keywords

record-keeping, records, **notes**, **security**, access, courts, writing, storage, **prejudice**

There are a number of issues around record-keeping which continue to grow in importance. The most fundamental of these concerns is whether there is an obligation to keep **records**. There is no consensus among counsellors in the UK on this issue, but the expectation that counsellors should keep records has grown. It is now rare to find a counsellor who does not routinely keep **notes** – however brief – of their work with clients. This chapter will consider the ethical reasons for keeping records, before exploring subsidiary issues about the **security** of records, access to records by clients, colleagues and the authorities, their content, and the question of how long records should be retained after the completion of **counselling**.

Is it Desirable to Keep Records?

The arguments in favour of record-keeping include:

- The process of writing records involves counsellors in organizing their thoughts and feelings. This is in itself helpful to the counselling because it enables counsellors to reflect systematically on what has occurred and plan for future sessions. In other words, the process of making records enhances the quality of the counselling.
- Records provide counsellors with an aide-mémoire for incidental details, such as the names of people mentioned by a client, and this then frees the counsellor to concentrate on issues raised by the client rather than recalling details from one session to another.
- Systematic record-keeping makes any changes in the client's material over a series of sessions more apparent. The process of recall by memory inevitably involves a degree of 'rewriting' the past in terms of a perspective rooted in the present. Written records produced contemporaneously with the counselling make any changes that have occurred during the counselling more visible. This provides valuable information to the counsellor, who may choose to share this knowledge with the client when it is appropriate.
- Systematic record-keeping provides evidence of the degree of care taken by counsellors in their work, which may be useful if a client makes a complaint against a counsellor to a professional body or begins legal action against a counsellor. It also protects against differences in memory between client and counsellor.
- As counsellors seek to be professional and credible with other professional services, they need to develop record-keeping practices that support them in performing their role and meet the public expectations of any professional for quality of service and **accountability**. This is regarded as an increasingly significant reason, which probably explains why most of the counsellors that we meet at workshops around the country have chosen to keep records.

The balance of practice has shifted towards an assumption that counsellors do keep records of their work unless there are good reasons for not doing so. Nonetheless there are ethical reasons not to keep records at all or only keep records for some clients for whom records are unproblematic. The arguments most frequently offered against record-keeping are:

- There are **problems** of ensuring that records are both secure and really confidential. For example, some counsellors may work in settings where burglaries are so frequent that it is difficult to maintain secure records. Community-based services operating out of converted buses or other forms of mobile premises have to consider the possibility of the theft of the entire counselling premises, including the records.
- Record-keeping may complicate **trust**-building with some clients. For example, counsellors working with clients who are vulnerable to legal prosecution (e.g. sex workers, illicit drug users and others) may have to take account of their clients' fear that the police or other authorities could seize any records.
- Record-keeping is time-consuming.
- Some counsellors are opposed to the possibility of clients acquiring a legal right to see records kept about them. Some counsellors, therefore, prefer not to keep records in order to prevent this eventuality.
- Some counsellors have reservations about creating records which may be demanded by clients for use outside the counselling relationship in legal actions against others. They hope that an absence of records will enable them to concentrate on the therapeutic relationship without having to consider how that work would be viewed in a court of **law**. If they hope that the absence of records will prevent them from being required to provide evidence in court cases involving a client, they will be disappointed. An absence of records means that the counsellor is more likely to be called in person as a witness because there is no other way of obtaining evidence. Where records exist, the counsellor may be permitted to provide a report of the relevant information based on the records or they may be required to submit all the records as an alternative to appearing in person.

It is clear from this summary of the case for and against the keeping of records that the arguments are, on balance, in favour of record-keeping by counsellors as a general standard of good practice. However, the argument in favour of keeping records can be countermanded by circumstances in which records cannot be kept securely or circumstances where the existence of records would deter clients and work against the public benefit of ensuring the availability of counselling on terms acceptable to clients. A client's attitude to record-keeping would also be relevant in individual cases. BACP's *Ethical Framework* states that:

> We will keep accurate records that:
>
> - are adequate, relevant and limited to what is necessary for the type of service being provided
> - comply with the applicable data protection requirements. (BACP, 2018b: 14)

Both the law and professional **ethics** require that clients have consented to records being kept. Ethically, this forms part of the client's full and informed consent. Legally, it is about citizens' **rights** to know about and exercise control over personally sensitive information that is being kept about them and to know the purpose for which it is being kept. When a client refuses to permit a counsellor to keep records, the counsellor is faced with a choice between continuing to see the client on this basis or refusing to see them unless some form of record can be kept. In my experience, most counsellors will attempt to establish why a client is so concerned about whether records are kept or not and attempt to adapt their practice to meet that client's needs. Some agencies will not see clients who totally refuse to permit any records at all.

Pause for Reflection

Do you keep records of your sessions with clients? If so, are these primarily for procedural purposes (i.e. because you are required to, or believe you are required to) or do you actively use them to reflect on your practice and in supervision so that they are **process notes** (a summary of a counsellor's personal feelings and psychological processes in response to a client's communications)? If yes, do you know what it is about your records that specifically facilitate this?

Security of Records

Once it has been decided to keep records, knowledge of their existence and the level of security with which they are kept become an aspect of the client's informed consent. There is a strong ethical argument that clients need to know these facts in order to be in control of the information that they decide to disclose to the counsellor; this represents an optimal standard. The minimum standard suggests that if clients are not informed about the security of records, they should be entitled to assume that records are kept with sufficient security to prevent them becoming known to people other than those authorized by the client. Counsellors who have taken this into account have adopted different kinds of procedures according to their circumstances.

The first line of defence against unauthorized **disclosure** is the physical security of the records. This would normally match the anticipated risks to the records. Locking records in a desk or filing cabinet will prevent casual inspection by anyone with access to the room in which they are kept, but this is inadequate against someone willing to force an entry as most desks and filing cabinets are easily broken into. Where forced entry is reasonably foreseeable, it may be more appropriate to keep the records in a safe. Keeping records in a physically secure container for hard copies and as electronically secure files on computers is a basic ethical requirement.

In addition to the physical security of the records, or sometimes as an alternative to it, some counsellors have adopted systems that ensure the anonymity of records. Four methods are frequently used:

1. The counsellor uses **codes** only they know to identify records. The code might be in the form of numbers or initials. No information is included within the records that could identify clients. This may be practical with small numbers of records but is usually impractical with larger quantities.
2. An alternative method is a split system of record-keeping. For example, personally identifiable information (e.g. name, address, contact numbers, names of significant others mentioned by the client) is kept on small file cards which can be readily removed from the premises by the counsellor, and especially overnight, from where the lengthier records of sessions may be kept. As each of these cards is numbered or coded and this is the only identification on the records, someone would need access to both the card and the record to obtain significant information about the counselling. The cards on their own only indicate who is receiving counselling but not the issues raised in that counselling. The records on their own merely contain the contents of the sessions but cannot easily be linked to identifiable people. Splitting records is only necessary where there are concerns about how securely records can be kept from unauthorized access. A single record system that is kept securely is much more efficient and **accessible** for routine use – especially in large or busy services.
3. Some counsellors work in settings where they are expected to make entries on agency records which are available to all authorized personnel within the agency, and may even be passed on to another agency if the client seeks their services subsequently. For example, counsellors in medical settings may be expected to make an entry on a patient's health record or, in social services, on a client's case file. Best practice in these circumstances usually involves the counsellor in negotiating an agreement with both the agency and their clients. Ideally, the agreement will permit the counsellor to make brief entries on the agency files and to keep separately more detailed records of the counselling process and any information which is personally sensitive to the client. These latter records would usually be treated as highly confidential and therefore access to them may be restricted to the counsellor and/or the client in routine situations. There is a legal precedent for this arrangement under the Code of Practice issued by the Human Fertilization & Embryology Authority (HFEA, 2008) as required by the

Human Fertilization and Embryology Act 1990. In this setting, it is usual for the offer of counselling to be recorded in the central records and the client's response to the offer. However, the counselling notes of individual sessions are stored separately and treated as confidential. Information obtained in counselling may be disclosed in certain circumstances, for example if it 'gives a team member cause for concern about the suitability of a person' to participate in fertility treatment. It is good practice to be clear with clients about how records are kept and the circumstances in which information might be communicated to other team members.

4. Increasing numbers of counsellors keep their records on computer. Such records can be protected by passwords and therefore be encrypted, which control different levels of access. Although the technology of computer records is different, the principles are much the same as for paper-based records, as detailed in the Data Protection Act 2018, the GDPR and the accompanying guidance. Counsellors also need to be mindful of where records are held: on a local hard drive of their computer, or in the 'cloud'. Many 'cloud' systems, such as iCloud and Dropbox, use servers outside of UK jurisdiction. It is a complex legal area, however, and most of the primary cloud services state compliance with GDPR requirements. There is an obligation for organisations and sole traders, which would include those in private practice, who process personal information to register with the Information Commissioner's Office and to pay a fee (see https://ico.org.uk).

Access to Records

The question of who ought to have access to records is frequently raised with regard to three situations. The first relates to situations where the counsellor is working in an agency in which the manager or employer is seeking access to client records; the second relates to a client's access to their own records; and the third relates to police access to files. It is useful to consider each of these separately because the ethical issues and legal considerations are different.

Access by employers

The demand for access to records by an employer is only possible when a counsellor has an employer. Counsellors working on their own in private practice are free from this particular concern. In some circumstances this may be a key factor in a client's choice of counsellor. Counsellors who have not clarified the status of their employer's access to records in advance of counselling, and are working without a corresponding agreement with their clients about access, are likely to find themselves in a difficult situation. The employer's and client's rights may be in conflict and both may hold the counsellor accountable.

The usual principle is that records made on materials provided by an employer or in the employer's time belong to that employer. However, the principles and law of **confidentiality** (see Chapter 10) suggest that there are restrictions on how an employer exercises that ownership. Ownership is not necessarily the same as unfettered control and access. Breaking a confidence without justification could create legal liabilities for a counsellor, even if the breach is to the counsellor's employer. A prudent counsellor will have established clear guidelines which are known to both the employer and the client about who will have access to counselling records and for what purposes in order to avoid conflicting responsibilities to the client and employer.

Access by clients

There is a strong ethical case for clients to be granted access to any personally sensitive information recorded about them in order for them to be reassured of its accuracy and to check that the information is consistent with the purpose for which it has been disclosed. In practice most clients will take records on **trust**, especially if their experience of the counselling is satisfactory. In some instances, however, a counsellor's **respect** for a client's **autonomy** over their records may be countermanded by a concern that granting access could destabilize the therapy and that access might be better delayed until that therapy is further advanced or completed. Such concerns can often be managed by negotiation (counsellors working in health settings may be able to enlist a doctor's authorization for restricting client access where the doctor considers such access would be seriously detrimental to the client's physical or mental health or condition, or indeed to any other person (see Data Protection (Subject Access Modification) (Health) Order 2000 5(1) implementing Data Protection Act 2018: this is probably the only exemption to a client's right of access likely to arise in counselling provided in a statutory service.)

Generally, data protection law lacks subtlety. It prioritizes a citizen's right to know personally sensitive information held about them so that they can challenge any inaccuracies and know for what purpose it is being kept and how it is being used. All the client has to do is make the request for access in writing, provide proof of identity if this is in doubt, and pay the required fee. However, the data holder should withhold from disclosure parts of the information from which another person could be identified, unless that person's consent has been given.

There is a rather odd legal exception to a client's right to see their counselling records, which is mostly restricted to non-statutory services. It is odd because there is no obvious ethical justification for this exemption. Indeed, it removes the right to see records in the very circumstances in which clients might be most concerned to see what has been recorded and how that information is being used and protected. The exception arises where the counselling records are held in an unstructured manual file. Such a file might be notes kept on paper and added to a cardboard envelope file in no particular order, so that finding a specific piece of information would require sorting and sifting through the file. Similarly, a file to which things are added in chronological order (e.g. the most recent item is added to the front or back of a ring binder) would be regarded as an unstructured file. The exact point at which a manual file turns from structured into unstructured is not precisely defined in law. It is determined by what is known as the 'temp test', that is, whether someone unfamiliar with the records, such as a temporary secretary, can easily find the information they are looking for by the way the record is structured (Mitchels and Bond, 2021). It follows that a file which is divided into sections is more likely to be a structured manual file to which the client has a legal right to see their own notes. In other words, the client's right to see records ceases in just those situations where they might be most concerned because the counsellor seems disorganized and unsystematic. A client has less right of access to a jumble of barely sorted papers than they have to a structured file (e.g. if the sections divide identification and contact details, session notes, discussions in **supervision**, correspondence etc.), so that someone could easily find a home address, notes of session 3 or discover when this client was last discussed in supervision.

From a client's perspective they would be best advised to see a well-organized counsellor, because not only will they have the benefits of that level of organization, they will also have the additional protection of access to the counsellor's records should it be desired under the data protection law. A client who sees a less well-organized counsellor may or may not suffer from their lack of organizational skills but will forego their right of access to the counselling notes. If a client obtains access to their notes and disagrees with what has been recorded because it is considered misleading or incomplete, the counsellor has a number of options. They may agree to some changes. Alternatively, they can record that there is a disagreement and record the client's version as an alternative version of events so that there are now two records of the same event.

Some counsellors will have legitimate concerns about granting clients access to their notes. Some will include personal notes about themselves and their own reactions as part of their process observations. A counsellor may then be concerned that these are too personally revealing to be shown to a client. Where such notes are integral to the counselling approach or methods, then the counsellor needs to ask why a client should not be entitled to see them. If they are too personal, could they be recorded in another way or held separately in a personal journal without any identifiable reference to the client? Clients are only entitled to access records which refer to them as identifiable persons because they are named, or their identity can be inferred from the information recorded. A client's notes are arguably not the place for a counsellor to be working through personal processes in depth, especially if they go beyond what is directly relevant to the client or if the counsellor wants to preserve their **privacy**.

Some psychodynamic counsellors have expressed concern about clients seeing records prematurely before transferences have been worked through and how this might disrupt the therapeutic process. There would be nothing to stop a counsellor asking a client to delay access, but that client would be entitled to insist on prompt access in the case of computerized and structured manual records. It is illegal to keep two sets of records relating to an identifiable client in order to grant access to one and keep the other away from the client. It should also be noted that the Data Protection Act 2018 does not permit withholding records from a client because they are damaging to the professional. A government department was ordered to disclose records that described their subject as a 'prat' and 'out-and-out nutter'.

The use of counsellors' records in court

What can a counsellor do if a client asks them to supply a report that will help them in a legal action against someone else?

Michelle has given birth to a severely disabled child and is bringing an action for medical negligence. Her counsellor is asked to provide a report about his client's feelings towards the child. The lawyers acting for the medical staff seek access to the therapy notes on which the counsellor based his report.

This, in broad terms, was the situation which Jakobi and Pratt (1992), as lawyers acting for the Psychologists Protection Society, were asked to consider. Counsellors may also be asked to provide reports following motor accidents, industrial accidents and in marital disputes.

Many counsellors are understandably reluctant to provide reports, appear as witnesses or supply case records on behalf of clients. To do so could be seen as a confusion of roles, with the counsellor being drawn into a public arena in ways that may compromise a client's autonomy or privacy. Counsellors may also feel that writing reports for courts is not part of their role and that they have not been trained in how to write these, in comparison to doctors and social workers who are usually more experienced in court work. It seems there is no way a client can compel a counsellor to produce a report on their behalf; the choice is the counsellor's.

However, refusing to provide a report may result in the client (or more likely the client's solicitor) requesting the court to issue a witness summons for the counsellor to appear in person to give evidence and for any records to be disclosed to the court. Often preparing a report that answers the solicitor's questions and protects the rest of the information is the better option and, in many cases, makes appearing as a witness unnecessary.

If a counsellor is asked to write a report on behalf of a client, Jakobi and Pratt (1992) recommend that a number of precautions are taken:

- The request for a report is likely to be made by the solicitors acting for the client. Technically, this can be treated as the client's consent to disclosure provided that the request comes from the client's own solicitors and not from solicitors acting for another party in the proceedings. However, it is sensible for a counsellor to see the client to ensure that they realize: that the production of the report could lead to a requirement for the disclosure of case records to the other party; that the counsellor may need to include sensitive information in the report; and that the client really is consenting to the production of the report (or client records) in full knowledge of what this entails.
- If a counsellor is asked to disclose records in addition to the report, this request should be refused unless either the client consents or a court order is made.
- If disclosure could cause serious harm to the client, then the counsellor should inform their solicitor so that an adequate explanation can be given for requiring disclosure. Again, through the client's solicitor, it may be possible to limit disclosure to matters that are highly relevant to the case or to restrict who sees the counselling records, such as a relevant expert. Alternatively, there may be other ways of obtaining the same information, perhaps by an expert examining the client independently.
- Sometimes it will be possible to request that an expert be appointed to examine the documents rather than have them considered in full in open court.
- If limitations on the disclosure of documents have been agreed, no reference should be made to the excluded material in court. Any limitations on disclosure will cease to have effect once the excluded material is referred to or read out in open court. A counsellor will need to bear this in mind if they are called to give evidence.

Once a client is engaged in litigation, a counsellor's notes are vulnerable to disclosure and use in proceedings. It is only in the most exceptional circumstances that a counsellor will be able to prevent disclosure. For a fuller account of the issues, see *Therapists in Court: Providing Evidence and Supporting Witnesses* (Bond and Sandhu, 2005) or seek legal **advice**. Whatever a counsellor does, they should not delay seeking advice until the last moment. This will make the situation very hard to resolve by using any alternatives that might have been available even a few weeks earlier.

Access by the police

The law places counsellors' records in a special category, which excludes them from the usual search warrant and substitutes a more demanding procedure before the police can obtain access to them. The legislation that established these procedures is historically significant as being the first to recognize formally the personal sensitivity of counselling records and grant them legal protection. The Police and Criminal Evidence Act 1984 requires a search warrant, which must be signed by a circuit judge instead of requiring only the more usual magistrate's signature, a less demanding procedure, to access files. This legislation is particularly interesting because it makes several specific references to counselling in its definition of 'personal records'. Personal records are defined in section 12 as:

> documentary and other records concerning an individual (whether living or dead) who can be identified from them and relating:
>
> 1. to his physical or mental health;
> 2. to spiritual counselling or assistance given or to be given to him; or
> 3. to counselling or assistance given or to be given to him for his personal welfare, by any voluntary organization or by any individual who –
>   i. by reason of his office or occupation has responsibilities for his personal welfare;
>   or
>   ii. by reason of an order of a court has responsibilities for his supervision.

Counsellors' records therefore belong in the same category as those of doctors, vicars and other spiritual leaders, social workers and probation officers, regardless of whether that counselling is paid or **voluntary**. Even if a circuit judge has signed a warrant, it is possible to go to the High Court to reverse this decision. In one case, the High Court ruled that an Old Bailey judge acted outside his powers when he ordered the Royal London Hospital to disclose someone's medical records to help in a murder investigation. This case demonstrates that counsellors can resist disclosing records to the police. An exception to the requirement for a warrant may arise if the police are searching for documents in order to detect or prevent terrorism under the Terrorism Act 2000. However, despite the sweeping powers seemingly given to the police under this legislation, they are required to exercise them 'reasonably'. It would be wise for counsellors to seek a lawyer's advice whenever they become aware that they are holding information which relates to a serious crime.

The Contents of Counselling Records

There are no fixed rules about what ought to be included in counselling records or how they ought to be written. Counselling records can vary considerably in style, from brief factual accounts which focus on what a client reported, to ones that include more of the counsellor's thoughts and responses. The guiding principle is that the type of record should be one that supports the therapy and enables it to be delivered to a reasonable standard of care. Another 'rule of thumb' might be to write notes assuming the client is sitting alongside you seeing what you are writing; some counsellors choose to actually do this and write records at the end of the session as a therapeutic and collaborative process with the client. A good record is written as close as possible in time to the events it records. Some counsellors will set aside 10 minutes between clients for this purpose. If we have any reason to think that a record might need to be produced for legal purposes, it is good to distinguish between what was directly observed, what the client said, and the counsellor's own responses or thoughts, as shown in the example below.

20 January 2020 Session 3

Bob arrived 10 minutes late, out of breath and looking rather flustered. He was more smartly dressed than for previous sessions and explained that a meeting with his boss at work had overrun and delayed him. He said that it had been his annual review. He had been dreading it – see previous session – but had decided to go in positively and make suggestions about how the administrative system that had been troubling him could be improved to everyone's advantage. He thought his boss was not interested initially but warmed to his ideas as he talked them through. This was not what he had expected. He said that he had expected his boss to dismiss his ideas out of hand. He had found the work on the similarities and differences between his boss and his father last week helped him to see them as different people who might react in different ways. He was pleased to be breaking a pattern of feeling silenced and deskilled. However, he is anxious about having to prepare a business plan for two weeks' time and has agreed to the next session being before this. I will monitor his anxiety, which he reports as 'half what it was when I first came to see you'. Noted that he did not mention his girlfriend or difficulties with her this time. As he left, I noticed that I was feeling uncertain about his motivation – between being liked or being successful? Explore further next time?

This would be a reasonably full record and appropriate if the counselling benefits from this level of detail and the counsellor has time to make the record. A shorter record of the same session might read like the one below:

20/1/10 Bob arrived late due to 'meeting with boss overrunning'. Bob thought meeting had gone better than expected. He said previous work on distinguishing his father and the boss had helped. Affirmed growing confidence. Consider exploring Bob's motivation at work next time.

Pause for Reflection

Which set of notes in the two examples given above do you prefer? What is the reason for your choice and is your preference for how you make notes influenced by the setting in which you work?

There is no single correct way of writing case notes. It still appears to be a neglected topic in basic training. Each counsellor has to develop a style that is sufficient to support the counselling but without being excessive in what is recorded. The primary purpose of good records is to support the work with the client. This will usually include a summary of significant content and processes. Other items to be included in the record are:

- any written and signed consents to all treatment;
- any written and signed consents to all passing of confidential information;
- all appointments, including non-attendance by client;
- treatment contracts (if used);
- up-to-date record of counsellor's reasoning behind decisions about significant interventions and general strategies;
- consultations with anyone else about the client;
- copies of any correspondence from the client or relating to work with the client;
- any instructions given to the client and whether or not the client acted on these.

Matters Not to Be Included in Records

Records ought not to include anything that could disrupt the therapy if seen by a client. **Prejudice** and abusive comments are to be avoided. Negative evaluations should only be included if they serve a therapeutic purpose; for example, a negative countertransference would be justified if it is integral to the therapy and a statement about the counsellor's internal processes rather than directly ascribed to the client ('I experience uncharacteristic boredom when Sue talks about her relationship with …', rather than 'Sue is boring about …'). Information about illegal behaviour, sexual practices or other sensitive information which may embarrass or harm a client or others is rarely appropriate for the record.

Giving careful consideration to what to include and exclude is good practice. What is included should be written with the possibility of the client seeing the record at a later date and the possibility that the records may be required for use in a legal dispute. However, the overall principle should be to write only what is useful for the therapy unless the record is known to be needed for other purposes and these purposes have been consented to by the client.

The Format of Counselling Records

Very little has been written about how best to structure counselling records. Houston (1995) recommends that counsellors keep the records in two sections. The first section should contain useful background information about the client and the contractual terms that have been agreed. She suggests the following headings:

1. NAME [probably coded] AND MEANS OF REFERRAL.
2. PRESENT CIRCUMSTANCES [Mrs A is 28, living since she was 18 with Claud. Works at Boots.]
3. HISTORY [Leave plenty of room to put in facts about her life and her ways of dealing with its events. These can be added to as the weeks go by. Noting the date can be informative here.]
4. REASON FOR SEEING ME [Has changed jobs three times in the last few months, and reports that finds working relationships with colleagues difficult, in contrast she gets on 'perfectly', her word, with family and Claud.]
5. MY HUNCHES [She said forcefully and out of the blue that she was not thinking of leaving work and having a baby. I guess she is. Longer-term work probably needs to be about her daring to acknowledge her own needs, and hopes for the future. To be explored sensitively.]
6. TIMES AND PAYMENTS [Tuesdays at 11 am, with 3-week break at Easter when she will be abroad. One month paid in advance, next payment due at next session.]

One way of establishing the contractual relationship with a client is for the counsellor to send them a letter or email after the first session that includes what has been agreed to between client and counsellor. The letter could be attached to this section, or the email printed off, as could copies of any subsequent correspondence.

The second part of the records would be the record of the actual counselling sessions. Houston suggests counsellors separate the factual account of what happened from their own personal responses and evaluations by using several vertical columns. The factual account of whether a client arrived on time, what was said and so on could be put down in the left-hand column. The commentary could then be written in a column to the right. There is a lot to commend this approach. At times when a counsellor has been seeing lots of clients, or when time is at a premium, they may use pre-printed forms or a standard computer template.

Use of Records in Counselling Supervision

Some supervisors will recommend or require that counsellors keep records and use these in counselling supervision. The process of writing notes helps a counsellor to sort their various responses to the counselling session and therefore helps them to focus their attention on important issues. It is agreed that this makes for a much better supervision session. This view is not universal, but it is gaining ground. Client consent should be sought for using records in supervision.

How Long Should Records Be Retained?

This is a difficult question to answer. Records may be relevant to present or future court proceedings, or to complaints, and so the time limits for legal proceedings

Name ....

Address ....

Contact tel nos: ....

Summary of counselling contract (e.g. frequency, duration, review periods, confidentiality, fees etc.):

....

....

Correspondence (attached) Code no*

....

....

* for split records only – NB no need to split records that can be kept securely

FIGURE 15.1 *Counselling records: client background information*

or complaints procedures may be relevant. The time limits for children and young people are different from those for adults (see Mitchels and Bond, 2021: Ch. 6). Sample record sheets are given in Figures 15.1 and 15.2.

Date: .... Time/duration: .... Code no* ....

Content: summary of client's narrative, behaviour, feelings and counsellor's interventions:

....

....

....

Process: any comments made by client about process, counsellor's observations and/or speculations about the process:

....

....

Notes for next session: e.g. any agreement about what the client or counsellor would do between sessions, issues to be raised during the session or for the counsellor to be aware of:

....

....

....

Issues for counselling supervision: ....

Notes about any correspondence or telephone conversations:

....

....

* for split records only

FIGURE 15.2 *Counselling records: record of each session*

The important thing is that a client should be aware of the amount of time that records are usually retained by a counsellor and agree to this. If a client wants their records retained for a longer period, this should be negotiated and agreed with the counsellor, or an alternative solution sought (perhaps that the records may be handed over to the client). In straightforward circumstances, where there are no other legal or professional considerations, the records could be destroyed any time after the end of the counselling relationship. One of the principles that informs good practice in record-keeping is that sensitive information should be destroyed when its usefulness has expired. A retention of one year might be appropriate where there is the possibility of a client returning.

However, where there are unresolved issues which might result in a complaint against a counsellor being made to a professional body or legal proceedings in which the records might need to be produced, a much longer period is required before the records should be destroyed. In the absence of any better guideline, seven to ten years would be appropriate, if this is both practical and the records can be kept securely. If any legal action involving a client is a possibility, it would be prudent for a counsellor to obtain legal advice about how long records should be kept, as the expiry time for initiating legal action varies according to the type of case. For a further consideration of how long to keep records, see Mitchels and Bond (2021).

Conclusion

It is now regarded as essential to good practice to keep records of counselling as these are part of a systematic and professional approach to counselling. Clients deserve this amount of care. Records are a very useful source of information that not only provide more accurate information than memory alone, but also support counsellors' professional accountability to clients and others with legitimate interests in their work as counsellors. As in so many other areas of society, there is a steady and accelerating movement away from paper records and communications with clients in favour of digital systems (see Chapter 11).

To access the online resources accompanying this chapter, please visit: https://study.sagepub.com/reevesandbond

16

Evaluation of Impact: Practice-based Evidence and Evidence-based Practice

Chapter Overview

This chapter considers the ethical case for counsellors being accountable to their clients and others. The use of **evidence-based practice** for determining the effectiveness of treatments and the basis for **accountability** and commissioning is examined. The ethical implications of current controversies over recommendations for the treatment of depression by **counselling** are explored before presenting the ethical case for service monitoring.

Key words

accountability, evidence-based practice, randomized controlled trials, **research**, monitoring

Evidence, evaluation and monitoring are not always the most popular topics with counsellors, many of whom tend to be more interested in working directly with people and their relationships rather than meeting the demands of evidence and **accountability**. Nonetheless, accountability is increasingly a part of what is necessary in the life of any health or social care professional in order to secure funding or attract new clients. Whether reluctantly or willingly, we are all being asked to look behind the positive claims we make for our services and to provide the evidence for what is being achieved. Every scandal in health and social care, and there have been many of them, undermines **trust** in the integrity of professionals unless that integrity can be backed up by evidence that demonstrates the **safety** and effectiveness of the services provided. Economic pressures on the best use of scarce resources have also increased the need for services to demonstrate that they are not only effective but are also better value than the available alternatives.

Accountability is an inescapable reality for most **counselling** services that are funded by either the public or commercial sector. Funders want to be certain that what they are funding is safe, effective and good value for money. Providing counselling in private practice for fees may escape the demands of accountability to an organization, but this is often replaced by an increased need to be directly accountable to clients. All successful counsellors, regardless of their setting, will have responsibilities and accountability to their professional bodies. Being accountable is an important aspect of being a successful professional and providing a valued service.

TABLE 16.1 *Ethical principles and accountability based on evidence*

Ethical principle	Reasons for accountability based on evidence
Being trustworthy	Being as professionally well-informed as possible about the possible benefits, risk of harm and costs to clients in order to be trustworthy
Respect for client autonomy	Having accurate and up-to-date knowledge to present to clients as the basis for their informed consent
Doing good	Being informed by the best and most relevant knowledge about how to offer effective and safe services to clients
Avoiding harm	Knowing what to avoid in order not to harm clients
Justice	Having the best available information to offer the most effective services to clients and to make best use of available resources
Self-respect	Being confident of the integrity, resilience and sustainability of the services we offer

The Ethical Case for Accountability on the Basis of Evidence

Professional **ethics** support the principle that we ought to be properly and appropriately accountable for the services we provide. Table 16.1 sets out the six ethical principles that underpin the *Ethical Framework* of the British Association for Counselling and Psychotherapy (BACP, 2018b: 9). Each principle represents a commitment to acting in a particular way, and this is an empty commitment unless a counsellor is willing to ask these questions:

- How do I demonstrate this principle in my practice?
- What is the appropriate evidence that will enable me to examine my delivery of this principle?
- What is the type of evidence that will be most helpful in identifying how to improve my service to clients and any other stakeholders in my work?

In practice, each of the ethical principles in Table 16.1 relates in different ways to some core questions:

- How effective is the service?
- How safe is the service? What are the potential risks and how is harm avoided?
- How do I know?
- To whom am I accountable for the answers to these questions?

For example, it would not be enough for a counsellor to say to a client 'Trust me, I am a counsellor' to demonstrate trustworthiness. It would be much better for them to be able explain clearly and briefly the type of therapy that is being offered, why it seems appropriate to this client, the benefits of what is being offered, and any risks of harm that need to be avoided. Without this information the client is deprived of information that will enable them to assess how much **trust** to put in a counsellor or the service they provide. Just as importantly the client will be unable to give informed consent, the hallmark of **respect** for client **autonomy**. Good practice in accountability strengthens a counsellor's ability to satisfy the principles of doing good or avoiding harm. A commitment to **justice** and **self-respect** will require a fair and honest evaluation of what is being offered in comparison to other possible services that might be available for the same types of **issues**.

Self-respect is much more secure when built on meeting the challenges of accountability based on honest assessments of strengths and weaknesses and a well-informed commitment to continue to develop and improve the service on offer. Resilience and sustainability are strengthened by appropriate accountability. In many ways all of this seems straightforward and perhaps a statement of the obvious to any conscientious counsellor. Unfortunately, the appearance of straightforwardness for counsellors quickly disappears when we ask them 'How effective is the service?' and 'How do you know?'.

Pause for Reflection

How do you know what you do as a counsellor is helpful to your clients? What measures of 'success' do you draw on to think about outcomes?

Evidence-based and Evidence-informed Practice

The **evidence-based practice** (EBP) movement started to become internationally influential in the 1990s as a scientifically robust way of distinguishing between interventions that worked and those that did not in both health and social care. The basic ideas behind EBP are very straightforward. It involves scientifically rigorous ways of systematically assessing the effectiveness of any type of treatment or intervention. It is motivated by a quest to fulfil the ethical principles of doing good and avoiding harm by providing scientific knowledge about the effects of different treatments. The most widely used method for analysing the impact of treatments or interventions is the randomized controlled trial (RCT). It involves providing a specified treatment to one group of people and comparing the outcomes with another group of people with identical characteristics who have not been given the treatment. All participants in the **research** have an equal chance of being allocated to either the treated or untreated group. The group who remain untreated are known as the control group. The characteristics and progress of the treated and control groups are measured in exactly the same way so that the effect of the treatment can be analysed statistically to high levels of accuracy.

RCTs are widely regarded as the 'gold standard' for researching effectiveness. Only a systematic review of several RCTs will usually lend more weight than a well-run single trial. So much evidential weight is given to RCTs that they effectively determine the clinical **guidance** offered by NICE (National Institute for Health and Care Excellence) or SIGN (Scottish Intercollegiate Guidelines Network). There are similar systems of guidance in the USA and Australia and many other developed countries.

Evidence-informed practice (EIP) adopts similar principles to those of EBP, but it draws on a wider range of evidence to support claims. Rather than being tied more rigidly to the 'gold standard' evidence of RCTs, EIP will draw on wider forms of evidence, such as single case studies, qualitative research and systematic reviews of previously published research, to draw together a picture of good practice *informed* by a wider range of materials.

It would be difficult to overstate the significance of the NICE and SIGN guidelines as they are having increasing influence on the commissioning and delivery of psychological services and only recommend therapies for which there is RCT evidence of effectiveness. The available evidence for counselling as an exploratory, non-directive or relational form of therapy is unfortunately relatively weak, with only a small number of studies showing some evidence of a short-term effect. This stands in marked contrast to cognitive behavioural therapies (CBT) where many more studies have been conducted and have demonstrated much stronger effectiveness in the treatment of depression and anxiety disorders. This is reflected in NICE guideline CG90 (2009) that only recommends counselling for people who have declined other treatments judged to be more effective. This recommendation comes with a significant caveat that the referrer should 'discuss with the person the uncertainty about the effectiveness of counselling' (NICE, 2009: s. 1.5.1.4). The latest working update to the guidelines for depression were unusually sent out for two sets of consultation following intense criticism with claims by many in the mental health field that they were not fit for purpose, drawing on too narrow an evidence-base and disregarding other research. The new iteration of the guidelines is still awaited at the time of writing with an expected publication date of 2022.

The SIGN guidelines simply state that 'there is insufficient evidence on which to base a recommendation' for counselling (Scottish Intercollegiate Guidelines Network, 2010). A lack of evidence points to 'not knowing' rather than knowing that something is ineffective or, even worse, harmful. The danger for counselling is that there are other therapies that have strong positive evidence. Practitioner experience is regarded as being a much lower level of evidence in the hierarchy of evidence. It falls below the threshold of evidence that influences clinical guidelines like NICE or SIGN's that determine decisions about what types of service to commission and fund in the public sector and increasingly in commercial sectors. The scientific **values** behind RCTs mean that they favour scientific evidence rather than the recommendations of practitioners, no matter how eminent. 'Eminence-based practice' is frequently compared unfavourably with 'evidence-based practice'.

Making sense of this state of affairs is not easy as there are many issues in play. As counsellors we tend to favour qualitative research and evidence as being most informative for our practice, which is mainly language-based. Many of us do not have the expertise or desire to interrogate or replicate the statistical analysis required in RCTs. Furthermore, there is a sense of unfairness that funding, for what are very expensive experiments, has been more readily available for research that investigates CBT than for counselling. There is a concern that research led by advocates of CBT may have been more conscientious in ensuring the quality of CBT practitioners than for counsellors. It is certainly the case that the leaders of the evidence-based movement have been very successful in advancing their case with policy-makers, and that this is now the leading approach internationally that seems set to become even more firmly established.

The ethical case for EBP is hard to refute, even when the conclusions are unwelcome or based on unfamiliar statistical techniques. It is a scientific methodology that directly addresses effectiveness, **safety** and efficiency more directly than any current alternatives. These are all substantial concerns in professional ethics. Like all science, the knowledge is provisional and may change with new studies or as the methodology is refined to support more sophisticated analyses. Cooper and Reeves (2012) argued that we would be mistaken to simply stand by passively in the hope that either RCTs will be superseded by methodologies more favourable to counselling or that guidelines will widen their evidence base to accommodate the qualitative types of evidence favoured by counsellors (even if clinical guidelines widen the evidence base, this will apply equally to all therapies under investigation so other therapies may still retain or strengthen their advantage.) Sanders and Hill (2014) have moved the argument on by providing an evidence-based approach to person-centred and experiential counselling for depression. Pybis et al. (2017) used counselling for depression and CBT data to compare the effectiveness of both models in the context of IAPT (Improving Access to Psychological Therapies) and were able to demonstrate similar effectiveness for treatment of depression that previous RCTs had not shown. This research has the potential to strengthen the argument for non-CBT approaches within IAPT.

Another possible way forward is to use the collective resources and expertise of our large professional organizations, anywhere in the world, to seek funding for RCTs that investigate issues relevant to counsellors and use the findings to inform how we develop our services. In parallel with promoting professionally relevant RCTs, it is equally useful to periodically undertake systematic reviews that gather all types of quantitative and qualitative evidence to investigate the impact of counselling in different settings or for particular issues.

Pause for Reflection

What are your views about the relationship between the delivery of counselling, and research? Would you consider yourself a practitioner-researcher, a critical consumer of research, or generally disinterested in research? How might this shape your work as a counsellor?

Evidence-based Service Development: Improving Access to Psychological Therapies

Improving Access to Psychological Therapies (IAPT) is an evidence-based development of services in England to address the shortage of services for people with psychological difficulties. In many ways, it is a development that represents the persuasive power of evidence-based policy and service implementation. IAPT started in 2006 with £3.7 million to set up pilot projects in Doncaster and Newham to work with people experiencing depression and anxiety. The service was substantially extended in 2011 to increase its geographical coverage and the types of problems addressed. This was all the more remarkable because the UK was in the depths of an economic recession which was leading to cuts in many other publicly funded services. Layard and others (Layard et al., 2007) championed a service, which later became IAPT, building the case by referring to NICE guidelines and arguing for the national economic benefits that an **accessible** service could provide.

The model for delivering the service is significantly different from how professions traditionally protect their **standards** by having a single point of entry to the profession to deliver a variety of levels of service, including some for which the professional may be over-qualified and therefore probably more expensive than would be strictly necessary. The aim is to respond quickly to demand with the lowest level of service appropriate to someone's condition in order prevent their condition developing and requiring more costly and demanding treatments. For clients, a stepped approach has the advantage of speed of response and ensuring they have the least time-consuming and intrusive treatment possible. For the agency there are efficiencies in how the service is delivered to the largest possible number of people at the lowest cost. The current service development priorities for IAPT are:

- *Expanding services:* To enable 1.9m adults to access treatment each year by 2024.
- *Focusing on people with long term conditions:* Two-thirds of people with a common mental health problem also have a long-term physical health problem, greatly increasing the cost of their care by an average of 45% more than those without a mental health problem. By integrating IAPT services with physical health services, the NHS can provide better support to this group of people and achieve better outcomes.
- *Supporting people to find or stay in work*: Good work contributes to good mental health, and IAPT services can better contribute to improved employment outcomes.
- *Improving quality and people's experience of services*: Improving the numbers of people who recover, reducing geographic variation between services, and

> reducing inequalities in access and outcomes for particular population groups are all important aspects of the development of IAPT services. (IAPT, 2020)

All this is ethically highly desirable when set against the ethical principles. Stepped care is not only better for clients in terms of matching services to their needs, it is also more beneficial by increasing the availability of services to people who would otherwise have no service. The stepped approach to delivering services arguably ensures that the greatest number of people are helped from the available resources by financial and personnel efficiencies.

Even when allowance is made for the ambition of the scheme and initial difficulties in introducing new services, some counsellors still have reservations based on their direct involvement. One reservation relates to the level of form filling required of clients as part of their therapy and monitoring of their progress. Some would argue that it is disproportionate to the benefits for clients. Too much data-gathering for monitoring takes the focus away from their needs. There is also a substantial amount of paperwork demanded from practitioners, and again some would consider this to be more onerous than helpful or even a substantial distraction (Mason and Reeves, 2018). There are regular deadlines for returns to the Health and Social Care Information Centre, which is the body responsible for the analysis of statistics about the delivery of IAPT.

The focus on statistics is invaluable to scientists wanting to understand the impact on cohorts of clients. It is also the language understood by NHS senior managers and the Treasury, who will want to assess value for money. The scientific paradigm offers the most valid and reliable ways of undertaking this type of monitoring and evaluation. Some counsellors appreciate the strategic purpose of this way of working. For others, the emphasis on quantification is alien. Many counsellors are more familiar with and have been trained to make qualitative assessments around individuals and their specific contexts. In the UK, perhaps more so than in the USA, counsellors are trained in and rely heavily on interpretive and postmodern paradigms which value different types of knowledge from the natural and biomedical sciences.

To see beyond the constraints of the individual and of particular contexts is generally viewed as a strength in science in the quest for general principles. A lack of active interest and a focus on the particular characteristics of different human experiences, life stories and their interpretation can be viewed as weaknesses from the viewpoint of personalized values and perspectives of counselling. The challenge is learning to live with differences, and possibly differences that challenge our assumptions about effectiveness. There is much to be learned from each other in the interests of developing the best possible services to clients. Ambivalence and differences of opinion ought not be a barrier to learning but a prompt to learning and investigating with greater energy.

Social Justice in Context

While the IAPT service has, in many ways, enabled more people to access the psychological therapies and has played a part in improving public awareness of talking therapies, its critics have suggested that insufficient numbers of people who access therapy through IAPT get better, or stay better, and that the type of evidence used to inform therapy development has been too narrow, reducing choice for clients and limiting innovation in non-CBT approaches. IAPT fundamentally speaks to what researchers call epistemology (the theory of knowledge) and ontology (the nature of being) and how positivism (objective measurement) still dominates the profession.

Monitoring and Professional Accountability

Monitoring services is less ambitious than scientifically proving effectiveness but is every bit as important. Monitoring involves having processes that assess the delivery of services and the identification of trends or issues which inform the development or improvement of the service or provide alerts to something going wrong. It is the basis of the professional management of any service and provides the information to support proper accountability that can be undertaken with integrity. The key questions are those with which we started this chapter:

- How effective is the service?
- How safe is the service? What are the potential risks and how is harm avoided?
- How do I know?
- To whom am I accountable for the answers to these questions?

The first task is describing the activities undertaken by the service in terms of numbers of clients seen, their main characteristics against gender and possibly age group, the range and average numbers of sessions received by clients, and the issues for which counselling is sought. In some services, this basic information needs to be matched against information about the numbers of counsellors involved or income. The aim is to give a meaningful overview of the service and its activities as the basis for answering the key questions.

The best way of gathering information about how a service is experienced is by gathering information from clients. It is their experiences and opinions about the service they have received that are essential to understanding the perceived effectiveness of the service. The absence of a control group means that it is not possible to measure effectiveness against scientific standards, but knowing the client's perceptions of the service is often more informative, operationally and ethically, about the quality of what is provided. The simplest way of doing this is an exit questionnaire. In practice, many services are more sophisticated than that. Many provide initial self-assessment forms and repeat many of the same questions at strategic points during the counselling or at its end to provide better quality insights into how the counselling has affected clients. For small services with limited resources, it may be appropriate to design a simple questionnaire or to have a standard set of questions to put to all clients orally at the end of their counselling. The alternative is to subscribe to an independent system which has the expertise to design and analyse the responses. The most widely used system in the UK is CORE, which not only provides forms free of charge but can also analyse the results in their own terms and against national benchmarks for a fee. Knowing how any counselling service performs in comparison to other services is probably one of the best starting points for understanding the strengths and challenges faced by the service.

Demonstrating the safety of services requires careful consideration of the risks to clients in the first instance, as well as to the people involved in working with clients such as receptionists and counsellors. A conventional way of doing this is periodically to review and identify risks and then to classify the likelihood of such an event occurring and the level of severity of the impact of that event if it were to occur. Something identified as having a high likelihood of occurring and severe impact would require immediate countermeasures to reduce both the likelihood and impact. For example, using computers without regularly updated **security** would represent a moderate to high risk of leaking client information that could have very adverse impacts on the service. The remedy is easy and should be implemented quickly.

Potential incidents that are unlikely to occur but would be considered as having a high adverse impact have to be considered carefully against the level of difficulty in preventing the risk. For example, the risk of one client attacking another with sufficient violence to cause serious injury would probably be assessed as relatively low in most services. However, the adverse impact would be high on the people concerned and the reputation of the service. Putting in place procedures and training to reduce the risk and ensuring effective responses when such a situation looks likely to arise would probably be a proportionate response. The arrangements to protect the safety of counsellors and other staff will also serve to protect the safety of clients in many services. In contrast, difficulty parking in many town centre sites is high but relatively low impact in terms of safety, but the potential for disrupted appointments and quality of client experience could be high unless clients are alerted to the issue and advised on travel and parking arrangements. The aim is to have responses that are proportionate to the risk.

Larger organizations may have risk registers in which risks are identified, assessed in terms of likelihood and severity of impact, and any actions taken are recorded. These registers are then regularly reviewed and updated. The same principles apply for smaller organizations, and even for single practitioners working alone, while regular reviews may not be recorded so formally but more significant concerns could be discussed in **supervision**.

Another aspect of safety is considering the likelihood of particular counselling techniques putting clients at risk and how this might arise and what countermeasures may be required to protect clients. Some of them can be identified in advance and good practice guidelines developed in much the same way as for other risks. However, some of the risks may be less obvious to the counsellor than the client, or the counsellor may not appreciate the client's experiences. Providing an effective way for clients to raise concerns and carefully considering the issues raised are usually the best way of enhancing client safety and improving the quality of their experience. Again, it is often easier to provide opportunities to raise issues in larger services than with counsellors working alone. In both cases it is ethically desirable not to become over-defensive in ways that discourage clients from raising concerns or leave them feeling blamed or pathologized. Keeping a record of any issues that have been raised and actions taken and periodically reviewing this record are another part of the monitoring process that helps to promote safety. Any service that experiences no issues being raised by clients has to consider the likelihood that everything is so perfect that there are no issues to be raised or whether there are hidden obstacles to clients raising issues. Services that routinely and systematically collect client feedback are much less likely to have significant issues passed over and unreported until they grow into major problems.

Accountability to Whom?

For counsellors working in agencies there is usually dual accountability, to a counselling supervisor and a service manager. Counsellors will usually be discussing issues around the safety and effectiveness of their work, and particularly around individual clients, with their supervisors. Some of the issues raised may have implications for the overall running of the service and therefore will be appropriately considered in staff or team meetings or raised with managers. It is usually the managers who take **responsibility** for overseeing the development of policies and their implementation with regard to effectiveness and safety. Depending on the type of organization, the managers may be working within a hierarchy of accountability ultimately reporting to a board of trustees or governors responsible for overseeing strategy and governance.

Sole practitioners are by definition more isolated and lacking in opportunities to share the responsibilities for monitoring effectiveness and safety than colleagues in an organization. The counselling supervisor may be the only person with formal responsibilities for oversight. Professional networks of sole practitioners who meet to discuss practice issues can be a viable way of keeping in touch with developments elsewhere, and provide a forum in which to report and discuss issues arising from monitoring the services provided.

The group of people who have most at stake in the quality of service providers are the clients. They are the primary stakeholders. Some services have developed ways of reporting back to client groups on the basis of 'You said … We did …'. Others have client groups that are more actively involved in developing and commenting on policy and practice at an earlier stage. However, the ethical commitment to protecting client **confidentiality** and **privacy** may make this inappropriate for some services. The challenge for all services of all types is how to engage with clients constructively on issues concerning effectiveness and safety.

The ultimate ethical function of all governance and monitoring activities is to enhance the quality of the service provided. The primary function of any service is to provide its frontline services. Everything else is secondary. Accountability and monitoring are essential but need to be proportionate to the benefits they generate for the frontline service or the viability of the service provided. This can involve difficult assessments of what are the desirable levels for accountability and monitoring. These need to be sufficient but not excessive. There is probably quite a range between these two extremes which will be viewed differently by different stakeholders. Professional bodies will often contribute to shaping the requirements and are the place for clients to raise concerns as a last resort, but it is so much better for all concerned to have good systems of accountability as close to the point of service as possible.

Conclusion

Being ethical requires counsellors to use both their therapeutic expertise and the best available evidence. Therapeutic expertise is acquired through training, continuing professional development, and carefully reflecting on the experience with clients. The best available evidence may come from a variety of sources. Where evidence from good-quality clinical trials with control groups is available, this needs to be taken seriously but not uncritically. In some cases, it may be considered right to investigate and adopt practices that have been independently assessed as effective. In others it may be possible to incorporate elements of effective practice into existing ways of working. In yet other cases, it may be clear that findings from EBP (e.g. NICE, NHS, counselling research) will not work with a particular client group or in a specific context. The ethical responsibilities to do good and avoid harm require carefully considered judgments for which the counsellor is willing to be accountable and offer reasoned explanations to colleagues and clients.

Another major source of information to be considered in deciding best practice can be derived from monitoring and reviewing what works well in a particular service. Depending on the service, this may be from the analysis of data in agency **records** and client feedback. Counsellors working in the UK will also have counselling supervision, which provides a further opportunity for careful consideration of all the available evidence to decide what is currently best practice and most likely to help clients.

When a general strategy for best practice has been selected for the counselling being offered by an agency or an individual counsellor, there are still judgments to be made with regard to individual clients and these start with the client. Sackett (1996), one of the most cited experts on EBP, was very conscious of the importance of ensuring that general principles should not override the specific needs and circumstances of individual patients or clients. He defined EBP as 'the conscientious, explicit and judicious use of current best evidence in making decisions about the care of the individual patient. It means integrating individual clinical [or counselling] expertise with the best available clinical evidence from systematic research' (1996). Making judgments that fit individual clients requires consideration of three elements:

1. Client values and experiences.
2. Counsellor expertise.
3. Best research evidence.

It is tempting to overstate the differences between EBP and EIP and other approaches that prioritize a counsellor's relationship with a client. Effective EBP still requires that clients are the primary focus, and building a strong counselling relationship with clients adds to its effectiveness. Client-focused approaches to counselling are not free of theory or knowledge. The ethical challenge for these approaches is to test the effectiveness of this theory and knowledge for their clients. Not to do so would have the effect of prioritizing the counsellor's beliefs and values over the interests of the client, which would be fundamentally inconsistent with any of the approaches to counselling built on client-centred values.

To access the online resources accompanying this chapter, please visit: https://study.sagepub.com/reevesandbond

Part IV

The Whole Picture

17

Ethical Problem Solving

Chapter Overview

Ethical **problems** and **dilemmas** are an inescapable part of being a counsellor. This chapter sets out a model for ethical problem solving and considers its application to three examples.

Key words

problems, **issues**, dilemmas, **responsibility**, action, evaluation

Whenever you are confronted with a problem or dilemma about **ethical standards**, it is useful to approach it in a systematic way. This maximizes the likelihood of reaching a solution which you are confident is the best possible outcome. This chapter contains a six-step process which is a development of an ethical problem-solving model derived from American sources (Paradise and Siegelwaks, 1982; Austin et al., 1990). It follows the basic principles of many problem-solving models used by counsellors with their clients but adapted to fit ethical problem solving. It has stood the test of time and anecdotal evidence suggests this model is often used by counsellors, perhaps in supervision, to consider situations they encounter in their work. It works best when it is taken as a basic framework and used to consider as wide a range of options as possible before making a decision.

Produce a Brief Description of the Problem or Dilemma

Making sure that we can produce a short spoken or written conceptual description of the main elements of our ethical dilemma is useful. Sometimes doing this reduces our confusion so effectively that the problem disappears. On the other hand, if the problem still remains we then have a good starting point from which to seek assistance and clarify the main **issues** to be considered. Struggling to define a problem is often a good indication that it is something that needs discussing with a **counselling** supervisor or another experienced counsellor. If it cannot be summarized, perhaps that is an indication that the problem is not clear yet. It is very difficult to make much progress in discussion of the issues until the main issues of the problem can be identified. It may be that some of the later steps will lead us to revise our description of the main points, but a short and clear statement of what these appear to be is a good starting point.

Whose Dilemma Is It Anyway?

This is a basic question that often casts a sharp light on the darkest of ethical **problems** in counselling. Counselling is an activity that requires careful monitoring of **boundaries** of **responsibility** in order to ensure that these are not becoming blurred. Chapter 6 suggested a useful way of approaching boundary issues, starting from the position that the counsellor is responsible for the process and methods used whilst the client holds responsibility for the outcome of the counselling. Often this general principle is very helpful, especially where the ethical issue concerns the relationship or work within the counselling. There may be rare exceptions to this principle where the counsellor considers that they hold some responsibility for protecting the client from **suicide** or protecting others. Protecting the client from harm is most likely to arise when the client is a young person or child, or a vulnerable adult. Protecting others may arise where the client threatens serious harm to another named person, especially if that person is also a client. It may be that there are good reasons for believing that a client is so distressed that they are incapable of taking responsibility for the outcome of the counselling and poses a threat to others. Fortunately, these situations are rare, and some counsellors may never encounter them. Nonetheless, it is a useful starting point to ensure that we have established the boundaries of responsibilities between ourselves and our clients.

The following scenarios are examples of issues relating to **ethics** and **standards** classified according to boundaries of responsibility.

Client's own ethical dilemma

Sheila decides she cannot face telling her partner that she has stronger feelings of attraction for someone else. She makes the decision to lie to her partner about the time she is spending with her new lover.

Trevor is feeling guilty about money he has embezzled from his employer. He had intended to pay it back but he has lost the money through gambling. He knows it puts the future of the business at risk. Should he tell his employer? (If the counselling is taking place in the work setting, it is likely that this would become a dilemma shared by counsellor and client.)

Counsellor's own ethical dilemma

Zoe is very wealthy and, having fallen out with all her close family, has decided that she wants to make a will bequeathing all her possessions to her counsellor. Her counsellor suspects that this is manipulation to win his support for Zoe's side in a family dispute. He also knows that if he accepts the bequest, it is likely that it will be suggested that he used his position of influence to persuade Zoe to make him a beneficiary. On the other hand, he would welcome being donated a large six-figure sum of money.

Frances has been talking in counselling sessions about her difficulties with someone who is already well known to her counsellor. Does he tell Frances that he knows the person she is talking about and risk inhibiting her, or does he stay silent?

Rachel has sought counselling from the student counselling service about whether to leave a course before its completion. Her counsellor knows that if one more student leaves this course it will be closed and the remaining students will be transferred to other courses. For one of the other very vulnerable clients, this could be disastrous as she sees this course as a lifeline. It could also have serious consequences for other students and staff.

The organization that employs the counsellor wishes to impose a restriction on the number of sessions he can offer to any one client. He knows that the maximum number of permitted sessions is unrealistically low for the majority of the clients he sees for counselling. What should the counsellor say to new clients who might be affected by the proposed policy? What should he do about the proposed policy?

(Continued)

Ethical dilemma shared by counsellor and client

Bill is unbearably stressed by his work, but he needs the income to support his partner and children. He decides that he must leave his employment but is feeling guilty about letting his family down. Therefore, he decides to lie to his wife and says that his counsellor has said that he should give up work. To add credibility to his deception, and without the counsellor's knowledge, he tells his wife that the counsellor is willing to see her and explain his recommendation. Bill's wife has arranged an interview with the counsellor. When she contacts him, the counsellor becomes aware that Bill has woven him into his deception and he will need to decide how far he is willing to share in the deception or distance himself from it while respecting Bill's rights as a client.

Susan seeks counselling about an eating disorder. She states that she is not receiving counselling or therapy from anyone else. The counsellor agrees to be her therapist. Several sessions later, Susan admits to having lied about not having another therapist. She had a prior agreement to work exclusively with someone else. She does not want to stop seeing the counsellor or the other therapist and values her work with the former. She feels unable to discuss seeing the counsellor with the other therapist.

One of the reasons for deciding at this stage who holds responsibility for the dilemma is that it may make all the subsequent steps in this model unnecessary. If a client has sole responsibility for the dilemma, it is most appropriate for the counsellor to explain the issue to the client and help that person make their own decision. Where there is joint responsibility, some clarification and negotiation with the client will usually be indicated. The stages that follow are particularly appropriate for the resolution of **dilemmas** that are primarily a counsellor's responsibility. On the other hand, the model is flexible enough to be shared, wholly or partially, with some clients in order to help them decide issues which are their own responsibility or joint responsibilities with the counsellor.

Consider All Available Ethical Principles and Guidelines

The aim of this stage is to become better informed about possible ways of resolving the ethical dilemma. It is helpful to review the ethical codes published by all the professional associations who hold a PSA accredited register in the counselling professions. Additionally, the guidelines produced for specific professional groups by the Nursing & Midwifery Council (NMC), the British Association of Social Workers (BASW), the various health and social care professions and the General Medical

Council (GMC) are highly relevant to counsellors working in related roles. They may also offer useful insights to counsellors in similar settings, but some caution may be indicated in assuming that they are directly transferable because of the different legal bases of specific professions and organizations. Some counselling services have developed their own codes and **guidance**, which can be very informative.

Some ethical issues cannot be decided without consideration of the **law**. Up-to-date publications may be useful but if the matter is complex or there is uncertainty about the law, it is strongly recommended a counsellor take legal **advice**. Some general questions that may come up are:

1. What actions are prohibited by law?
2. What actions are required to be performed by law?
3. What rights and responsibilities does the law protect?

In the absence of any relevant guidelines or definitive legal advice, a counsellor may find they need to consider the issue on the basis of general ethical principles. For example, BACP (2018b) uses six principles that underpin its *Ethical Frameworks*:

- *Being trustworthy*: honouring the trust placed in the practitioner.
- *Autonomy*: respect for the client's right to be self-governing.
- *Beneficence*: a commitment to promoting the client's wellbeing.
- *Non-maleficence*: a commitment to avoiding harm to the client.
- *Justice*: the fair and impartial treatment of all clients and the provision of adequate services.
- *Self-respect*: fostering the practitioner's self-knowledge and care for self.

In counselling, the first principle is especially important and will often prove decisive, particularly if it is possible to act in ways consistent with satisfying one or more of the other principles.

At the end of this stage counsellors would hope to be clearer about which goals are ethically desirable. This will then provide an orientation and some criteria for choosing between possible courses of action.

Identify All Possible Courses of Action

This stage is an opportunity to brainstorm all the possible courses of action that will achieve the ethical goals identified in the earlier stage. Some courses of action will seem highly probable ways of resolving the dilemma. Others may not seem feasible. However, it is better not to discard the less realistic ideas too readily because sometimes these will contain the basis for an original approach or new insight.

Select the Best Course of Action

A former Chair of the American Association for Counseling and Development (Stadler, 1986a, 1986b) proposed three tests for a chosen course of action that have their origins in moral philosophy and have stood the test of time: these are composed of a series of questions:

- *Universality*
  - Could the chosen course of action be recommended to others?
  - Would I condone the proposed course of action if it was done by someone else?
- *Publicity*
  - Could I explain my chosen course of action to other counsellors?
  - Would I be willing to have my actions and rationale exposed to scrutiny in a public forum (e.g. at a workshop, in a professional journal or newspaper, or on radio/TV)?
- *Justice*
  - Would I do the same for other clients in a similar situation?
  - Would I do the same if the client was well known or influential?

If we find that the answer 'no' applies to any of these questions, we may need to reconsider our chosen outcome. A final step in identifying the best course of action may be to check whether the resources are available to implement what is proposed.

The aim of this stage is to make an informed choice between all the possible courses of action identified. Consideration of guidelines and the law in the previous stage will be useful but may not be decisive. Asking these questions can therefore usually prove very informative.

Evaluate the Outcome

After we have implemented a course of action, it is useful to evaluate it in order to learn from the experience and prepare for any similar situations in the future:

- Was the outcome as I hoped?
- Had I considered all relevant factors with the result that no new factors emerged after I implemented my chosen course of action?
- Would I do the same again in similar circumstances?

Examples of Ethical Problem Solving

Below are some examples of how this model of ethical problem solving might work in practice. The first two raise the issue of dual relationships. Examples 3 and 4 pose what participants in training workshops often consider to be amongst the most difficult ethical dilemmas: child protection and confidentiality. The aim of these examples and of Example 5 is to illustrate how the model works rather than suggesting that the conclusions are necessarily right. The same model can be used but produce different conclusions.

Dual relationships

Example 1

A counsellor is approached by Pam, the teenage daughter of a friend, who asks him to offer her counselling. The counsellor hardly knows Pam but it is apparent that she is emotionally troubled and has dropped hints about not eating properly. Pam is insistent that from her point of view he is ideal as a counsellor as he is neither a stranger nor too close. She turns down any suggestion of seeing anyone else. It has taken her months to pluck up the courage to speak to the counsellor. The counsellor checks with her mother who is a friend of his. She is supportive of the idea and offers to pay whatever is the usual fee. The counsellor feels her friendship matters to him.

Example 2

Kareen is very pleased with the help she has received from her counsellor. She would like her daughter to see the same counsellor.

Pause for Reflection

For each example, use the ethical problem-solving model to identify the issues that the counsellor ought to consider. What ethical issues do these requests raise? How ought the counsellor to respond?

We have outlined below a commentary on the scenario in Example 1 to show what an ethical problem-solving approach might look like.

The first step is for the counsellor to produce a brief description of the dilemma. The main elements are:

- Divided loyalties if the counsellor takes on Pam as a client between her interests as a client and his friendship with her mother. What if Pam's difficulties involve her relationship with her mother or perhaps abuse within the family?
- As a subsidiary issue, the management of confidentiality in relation to the mother, also a friend. The counsellor suspects that neither Pam nor her mother understands some of the potential complications of what is proposed.
- A further subsidiary issue: the payment for counselling by someone other than the client when there is uncertainty about that person's role in the client's problems. This could be considered once the other issues have been resolved.

The second step is to consider whose dilemma is it anyway? As it is presented, Pam and her mother are in agreement and the onus is on the counsellor to accept or reject the role of counselling Pam.

The third step is for the counsellor to consider all the relevant available codes and guidelines, especially those that relate to his registration as a counsellor or produced by his professional body. The BACP *Ethical Framework for Good Practice in the Counselling Professions* places responsibility on counsellors for determining the potential beneficial or detrimental impact of dual relationships on clients, and that they should be readily accountable to clients and colleagues for any dual relationships that occur (BACP, 2018a). Similar requirements have been stated by other national bodies. Some models of counselling are more open to this type of dual relationship than others. For example, it might be more problematic maintaining professional distance in a psychodynamic approach than in a person-centred or cognitive-behavioural way of working. The situation raises the question of whether the overlapping and pre-existing relationships are avoidable. The possibility of referral has been considered but this is unacceptable to Pam. There is also the additional requirement to explain the implications of maintaining boundaries to Pam, and perhaps secondarily to her mother. In what ways might the boundaries become blurred? For the client, it is a potential dual relationship with Pam as 'counsellor' and 'mother's friend' simultaneously. A secondary issue is the potential dual relationship with Pam's mother as 'daughter's counsellor' and 'friend'.

Ethical attitudes to dual relationships have relaxed on both sides of the Atlantic, from an instinctive prohibition to placing a great deal of responsibility on the counsellor for determining the therapeutic impact of such a relationship and ensuring that the benefits outweigh anything detrimental (Corey et al., 2003; Syme, 2003; Gabriel, 2005; Sommers-Flanagan and Sommers-Flanagan, 2007; Amis, 2017).

There are no apparent legal constraints. Therefore, the next step is for the counsellor to consider all possible courses of action. These will include:

- refusing to take Pam on as client, stating the reasons;
- offering a 'white lie' for not taking Pam on (e.g. too busy, not working with teenagers);
- agreeing to see Pam but only once she understands the potential conflicts of interest and has explored how she wants the counsellor to deal with any issues relating to her mother;
- agreeing to see Pam, but for as long as the counsellor is doing so minimizing contact with her mother, and having a clear agreement with both Pam and her mother about confidentiality and what may be communicated;
- accepting the risk of losing a friend by seeing Pam;
- seeing Pam for a fixed period with a review at which the possibility of referral or continuation will be considered.

The final stage is for the counsellor to choose a possible course of action. This choice will depend on the exact circumstances of the situation and his assessment of the possibility of maintaining clear boundaries and the likelihood of being able to help Pam. Perhaps it would be preferable to decline this dual relationship on ethical grounds given that it is likely that Pam will have issues relating to her mother, which she will need to explore and resolve for herself in the process of overcoming her eating disorder. The existing friendship with her mother is likely to complicate this process both for Pam and her counsellor. If there were any role to take on, it would be to assist Pam in finding a source of help which she considered acceptable and perhaps offering to be present to introduce Pam to her counsellor or therapist before they start working together. It would be important to be quite firm about the ethical undesirability of taking on the role of counsellor in these circumstances, and being quite active in giving Pam information that could assist her search for an alternative source of help. He would be unlikely to charge any fees for providing this information, so the subsidiary problem would not arise. However, it is often an issue when seeing young people so it is worth considering.

The third-order issue of payment of fees by someone other than the client is often tricky, especially if a client's relationship with the person making the payment might be an issue in the counselling. It is possible that the client will experience a sense of guilt about using counselling to explore difficulties with the benefactor, and may avoid this subject. The counsellor may experience similar inhibitions. This arrangement therefore may be contrary to an ethical commitment to respecting the client's autonomy, which implies actively promoting the client's control over her life. Several alternatives exist here:

- reducing the fees to a level where the client can afford direct payment;
- the client making a contribution towards the fees paid by someone else;

- suggesting that the money for fees be given as a gift to the client, who takes responsibility for managing payment to the counsellor.

Any of these arrangements would be preferable to direct payment by the mother, which might further confuse an already difficult set of dual relationships. It might be preferable to reduce fees to a level the client can afford directly. This provides the best way of placing the client in control of the counselling relationship. However, if this is not feasible, the client may make a contribution to the fees and take responsibility for managing the payment of fees.

Child protection and confidentiality

Example 3

James, a 19-year-old client, is seeing a counsellor for help with friendship difficulties and low self-confidence. After a few sessions, he hints that he is being sexually abused by an adult but asks for a promise that the counsellor will keep what he says confidential before he is willing to say more. Later he reveals that his abuser may be abusing younger relatives but he insists on having his confidentiality protected.

Example 4

Frank is a young adult who is very insistent that he wants his confidences about his own experience of being abused by his step-father and the possible risks of abuse to his younger step-brother, Alfie, is kept confidential.

Pause for Reflection

Using the ethical problem-solving model, for each example, 3 and 4, what are the main issues you would consider to help you reach a decision? How would you implement your decision in ways that are consistent with the values of counselling?

This is an increasingly common situation for counsellors. It is a welcome development that people are more likely to seek help for the consequences of being abused and that there is greater public awareness of abuse and neglect. It is so much better to be able to talk than suffer in silence. A commitment to prevent and detect child abuse has steadily grown in importance in public policy. It is also the case that child protection services have greatly improved, but they vary from area to area. No matter how much local services have improved, a young person who has experience of being abused is likely to be wary because they have direct experience of the harm that humans can inflict on each other. In each of these examples, a young adult has taken the first cautious step in putting his trust in another person, a counsellor.

In real life, the counsellor will have some sense of how far this is trust based on a developing sense of each other or whether James for example, is seeking help out of desperation to escape an intolerable situation. Where it is the former, the counsellor will want to honour the trust that is being offered. Where James is beginning to talk out of desperation, the counsellor will be aware of his vulnerability and emotional pain. It is often the case that communications about being abused are usually prompted by a mixture of hoping to be able to trust someone and the desire to get out of an intolerable and painful situation. Being ethical in such circumstances is a matter not only of professional integrity but also of helping someone to begin to trust again.

The dilemma in this case arises from James's request for confidentiality. Increasingly, counsellors will feel a moral obligation to act to protect vulnerable young people from abuse in relationships where they are systematically disempowered, or counsellors are under actual legal obligations arising from a contract of employment to report current child abuse. How should a counsellor respond to James's request for a promise of confidentiality? The tension is between working in ways that build a client's confidence and trust to counteract an abusive relationship or to intervene and attempt to build that relationship afterwards. So much will depend on:

- the counsellor's sense of the young person and what they will tolerate or, preferably, actively support and the significance of forming a therapeutic relationship;
- an assessment of the overall best interests of the young person concerned;
- the severity of the abuse and the imminence of any repetition;
- any known risks to other young people being abused by the same perpetrator;
- the legal framework in which the counsellor is working, particularly the contract of employment and whether or not the service falls within statutory children's services (see Mitchels and Bond, 2021).

These sorts of situations are difficult to predict, and it is unwise for counsellors to promise total confidentiality. It is generally much better if they actively consider how to remain respectful and trustworthy for the young person concerned. In some cases, this may require reporting concerns about current abuse to a client or others whilst being supportive of that client. This may mean being actively involved in the referral process and possible case conferences following a disclosure to the authorities. The fear for a counsellor is that breaking a client's confidentiality before they feel ready to do so will destroy the trust they have placed in the counsellor and be experienced as an additional betrayal. As services and procedures for investigation are developing rapidly in this field, it is sound practice for counsellors to seek the advice of specialists in child protection. Such discussions can often be opened in ways that protect the anonymity of the client until it is clear that either the client is ready to consent to disclosure or it is considered that the seriousness of the situation requires immediate disclosure. For the ethical basis of confidentiality, see Chapter 10.

Working online

Example 5

Emily is working with a client who is moving to another part of the country. Her client would like to continue working with her online. Emily is unsure whether this is a good idea, therapeutically and ethically.

Pause for Reflection

What are the issues that need to be considered and how ought Emily to resolve them in her practice? How might she use the ethical problem-solving model in supervision?

Some counsellors will make a strategic decision to offer their services online in combination with, or as an alternative to, working face to face, particularly in light of adapting to the COVID-19 pandemic. The advantage of making such a major decision is that it justifies a major investment of time and resources to develop a service operating at the appropriate therapeutic and ethical standards. Changing one's way of working for one client requires meeting the same therapeutic and ethical standards, but considering the level of commitment to make this achievable and whether it is desirable is a more complex problem to solve. Discussing the issues in supervision is a good point for counsellors to start.

In broad terms the ethical issues of working online are remarkably similar to working face to face, but the use of digital technology may introduce new twists in how issues arise and how they may be solved. This will become readily apparent from the start of the ethical problem-solving model.

Whose dilemma is it?

At this point it is the counsellor's. She has a decision to make and communicate to her client.

Consider all the available ethical principles and guidelines

As was discussed in Chapter 11, there is a rapidly growing body of useful literature and online resources to assist the counsellor and her supervisor in identifying what the key issues might be. In a rapidly changing field drawing on some of these resources would be highly advisable.

Others may be selected because they are still viewed as authoritative guidance or have been issued by the professional bodies to which the counsellor is accountable. The many different issues that will need to be considered suggest that it will be advisable for a counsellor to compile a list (see Figure 17.1).

Identify all possible courses of action

At the top level, there are two potential courses of action. The counsellor may accept or decline the client's request. However, these two options may depend on a second level of decisions about what sort of online contact the client is wanting and the practical and ethical issues associated with the selected methods of communication.

Select the best course of action

A great deal will depend on the counsellor's assessment of the suitability of the client for working online and her own desire to take on the challenges of working online. For someone who has a suitable client, good technological knowledge, access to relevant training or support and an appropriate supervisor or others to consult, the possibility of starting with a motivated and willing client may seem an attractive option. Any significant doubts on any of these points suggests that it would be

1. *Type of communication to be used.* These include texting, Twitter, Facebook, LinkedIn or other social media, email, video conferencing by Skype, Zoom, Microsoft Teams or purpose-designed secure platforms for counselling.
2. *Balancing security against accessibility.* Factors that will influence this balance will be:
   - the client's views on the sensitivity of what they intend to discuss;
   - what is technologically and financially possible;
   - the counsellor's assessment of the risks professionally;
   - selecting the best supported system;
   - availability of training in the technological and therapeutic methods to be used.
3. *Adapting the contract from face-to-face to working online by*:
   - establishing acceptable alternative means of communication in case the preferred method of working fails, for example landline or mobile phone, texting or email;
   - ensuring that both client and counsellor update and maintain the security and functioning of their respective links;
   - stating how work will be charged and paid;
   - securing confidentiality requirements for any additional technological support or therapeutic supervision.
4. *Other issues*:
   - insurance (most insurance companies require notification);
   - registration with the Information Commissioner's Office (or equivalent) and data protection requirements;
   - if working across national boundaries establishing which legal system applies, thus avoiding infringement of professional regulations requirements.

FIGURE 17.1 *List of issues to be considered when moving to online counselling*

better to decline the request. It would be hard to answer positively the three tests of universality, publicity and justice outlined earlier in the chapter.

Evaluate the outcome

If the counsellor decides to proceed with adequate preparation, the nature of the problem changes: it is no longer hers alone. Deciding the best way of working will mean adequately informing the client about the issues both counsellor and client need to be aware of, and developing a joint approach to distributing responsibility and risk between them will be necessary to establish an ethically secure therapeutic relationship. Both parties will be on a steep learning curve so regular reviews will be desirable. The degree to which it is considered appropriate and the client is willing to engage in a new professional enterprise, possibly on an experimental basis, will be decisive.

If the counsellor declines her client's request for online working, then she may want to consider whether she feels any responsibility for helping her client find suitable counselling in her new location or another source of online counselling.

Conclusion

Ethical dilemmas occur on a daily basis in counselling. Fortunately, most of them will be on a manageable scale after careful reflection. Many are more likely to be of the order of considering whether to refer a client, choosing what to discuss in counselling supervision, or deciding whether your client has consented to your proposed course of action. Resolving ethical dilemmas requires thought, knowledge and feeling, and may also demand the courage to make and sustain decisions. Carroll (1993) has likened resolving ethical dilemmas to general problem solving and argues that it is a process in which counsellors can become more skilled with training.

The model of ethical problem solving offered here is not definitive, but it is intended to be useful in everyday counselling. It is sufficiently flexible to incorporate insights from any of the six sources of professional ethics outlined in Chapter 3. Ethical dilemmas are usually a professional and personal challenge, but they can also be a source of new learning for the counsellor (Bond, 1997) when that learning is shared with the profession as a whole. Regular use of this model assists in counsellors maturing in their judgment and wisdom (Carroll and Shaw, 2013). Feedback from counsellors who have used this approach to ethical problem solving in supervision has been very positive.

Pause for Reflection

In a busy professional life, it is tempting to overlook problems that are successfully solved and to keep the available attention on problems yet to be solved and those that are hard to resolve. How do you keep a balance between problems solved and those that are unresolved? Are you able to apply learning from resolved problems to those pressing to be solved?

To access the online resources accompanying this chapter, please visit: https://study.sagepub.com/reevesandbond

18

Implications for Practice

Chapter Overview

This chapter considers the implications of **counselling** becoming a mainstream professional activity and how that requires reinvigorating our ethical commitment. 'Putting our clients first' is one way of achieving this. The distinctive elements of counselling practice that support us in achieving this goal are reviewed. The chapter closes with consideration of the role of ethical **mindfulness**.

Key words

professional, **regulation**, scandals, **supervision**, ethical mindfulness

The ethical context of **counselling** continues to change in ways that require counsellors to reconsider established ethical practice. Changes tend to be progressive and incremental, moving at the pace of social change, but may in some instances require substantial jumps to keep up. One such jump is in progress.

Changing Ethical Contexts for Counselling

Internationally there have been considerable changes in how counselling positions itself as a professional activity. What was once a radical social movement has increasingly joined the mainstream and slowly moved to a regulated position across the USA by legally protecting who is entitled to call themselves 'counselor' or offer 'counseling services'. The UK has adopted a different model of **regulation** through accredited **voluntary** registration which works rather like a quality kite mark. The debates around voluntary versus statutory regulation continue in many territories, with strong feelings on both sides of the debate. These positions have been further contextualized in the UK with the second consultation of SCoPEd, as discussed more fully in Chapter 8.

Regardless of whether counselling is regulated or not, there is increasing emphasis on the trustworthiness of the counsellor and, in almost all contexts, an increased expectation that counsellors ought to be accountable to their clients and other key stakeholders in their services. Whilst there is, and probably always will be, a concern about protecting client **confidentiality** and **privacy**, this is increasingly being moderated with regard to professional communications between fellow professionals on a confidential basis to enhance client **safety** and the quality of services provided. Counselling could be said to be maturing as a profession in terms of developing a sense of collective **identity** that is often stronger than the tensions between various approaches to counselling. The popularity of counselling with many people as an intervention to help with bereavement, trauma, mild to moderate mental and physical health **issues**, relationship **problems**, developmental and transitional issues is testimony to how counselling has advanced. However, as counselling has grown in volume of activity, so have the challenges of ensuring a shared understanding of **ethical standards** and that all services offered to the public meet minimum **standards**. Regardless of national organizations or type of regulation, the ability to establish and sustain standards will depend on creating a professional **culture** that encourages scrutiny and **accountability** between counsellors and appropriate collaboration and accountability when working with colleagues from other professions.

Putting the Client First

Counselling has much in common with other professions. Each profession has distinctive concerns to sustain its knowledge base, advance practice, secure employment and create career pathways. Counselling is still in a process of catching up with more established professions in health and social care in most countries. It is easy to lose sight of the primary purpose of professional **ethics** at such critically important moments in any profession's development. Professional ethics and the development of **codes**, procedures and organizations are all essential features of established professions. Counsellors have strong interests in advancing their claims to being a profession and rightly invest their time and resources to satisfy the requirements of being professionals. However, this is not the primary purpose of professional ethics.

The primary purpose of professional ethics is to put the client first in the competing claims for any professional's attention. Counsellors are no exception. We have had a salutary reminder of this in the UK as so many of the closely related professions involved in health and social care have been affected by a long series of scandals that have had serious consequences for clients and patients (see Table 18.1).

TABLE 18.1 *Health and social care scandals in the UK*

Types of scandal	Selected examples
Failed child protection	Numerous tragic cases where professionals failed to protect young children from lethal neglect or abuse by parents/carers in over 200 cases from Maria Colwell (1973) Victoria Climbié (2000) Baby P (2007) to Jamie Kightley (2012) – failure to share information between services has been a recurrent fault. Gangs of mostly young adult males have groomed and sexually abused vulnerable teenagers in Rotherham (2010) and other cities. Police and children's services failed to intervene effectively – even when help was sought by victims or their families. Jimmy Savile was able to use his celebrity DJ status and charitable fundraising activities to abuse over 60 vulnerable young people and adults in hospitals and elsewhere from 1962 to 2009. He abused almost in 'plain sight' with police and other staff seemingly feeling unable or unwilling to act on suspicions.
Abuse of young people by professional staff	Children and young people were systematically sexually abused by staff in north Wales children's homes (1974–1990) and elsewhere.
Serious neglect of highly dependent patients	Serious failures in basic care and neglect resulted in possibly several hundred premature deaths of elderly highly dependent patients in Stafford Hospital (2005–2009).

(Continued)

TABLE 18.1 *(Continued)*

Types of scandal	Selected examples
Poor or inadequate medical treatment	Heart operations on young children in Bristol Royal Infirmary (1984–1995) led to unnecessarily high death rates. This was thought to be due to a culture that encouraged ambition and professional competitiveness over concern about patient safety. A senior surgeon in Solihull Hospital was permitted to continue to use inadequate or outdated operation techniques from 1998 to 2010 for breast cancer in spite of concerns of colleagues and managers. Failure to intervene resulted in recalling about 500 patients for health checks and the General Medical Council suspended the surgeon in 2012.
Unethical retention of children's organs	During the Bristol Heart Hospital inquiry a witness revealed the unauthorized retention of about 850 children's organs for research at Alder Hey Children's Hospital from 1998 to 1995.
Murder of patients by medics and nurses	There have been a small number of cases of health workers who have used their professional role to kill several patients. Beverly Allitt was convicted for murdering four children and attempting to kill three others in 1991 by injecting overdoses of insulin. Dr Harold Shipman was convicted of murdering 15 patients between 1995 and 1998 and is suspected of murdering many more. He successfully concealed the theft of drugs used to kill patients and issued false death certificates from other health professionals by largely working alone in a system with weak monitoring of patient outcomes and inadequate accountability.

What is particularly troubling about these scandals is that professionals who tried to raise legitimate concerns at the earlier stages in things going wrong were often been ignored, silenced or bullied. The dominant culture has been to protect the reputation of the service or the profession rather than protect the client. It is such a common response across different types of scandal, different professions and settings that it appears to be deeply embedded in the prevailing culture. Culture is probably one of the most complex and powerful influences on behaviour. It is also one of the most difficult to change once it is established within an organization or across organizations.

Attending to the client's safety and wellbeing

This means putting the client at the heart of all we do and being particularly attentive to their **safety** and wellbeing whilst working with them. It also means that where there are choices to be made, careful consideration must be given to the impact on clients. This does not exempt us from difficult decisions. We will still find ourselves having to decide between the needs of individual clients and the best ways of providing services when demand outstrips supply. This is always difficult when the available resources are limited or need to be rationed. This is a situation where good practice encourages shared communications between managers, counsellors and their supervisors to reach the fairest possible decision.

Putting our clients first raises the issue of how to communicate our ethical commitments as effectively as possible to clients. Most codes and ethical frameworks are too lengthy and complex as documents to be of interest to any but a minority of clients. Some professions in the UK have been experimenting with succinct statements of key ethical 'duties'. The simplicity and shortness of this way of expressing ethical commitments appear to be well received by clients. This is an approach that seems to have potential for counselling as a way of communicating our ethical commitments to clients, colleagues in other professions, and ourselves.

Recognizing the significance of trust and being trustworthy as a substantial ethical challenge that directs our attention to specific issues

'**Trust**' is a word that often passes unnoticed in ethics as being too vague and imprecise to carry substantive ethical content. It can be used as little more than a feel-good factor that elicits positive responses. However, trust can also carry substantial ethical content when its implications are considered more carefully, especially in contexts like counselling where the quality and integrity of the relationship carry such ethical significance. Trust can be defined in ways that address areas of client vulnerability and express the counsellor's awareness and commitment in responding to them in ways that promote a client's wellbeing. Many relational challenges arise from the difference and inequality between client and counsellor. They can be particularly acute at the beginning of a counselling relationship when the client may feel vulnerable to being diminished, blamed or scapegoated because of differences or feel disempowered by being in the position of seeking help from someone who is assumed to have the expertise and associated authority of a healer. These relational challenges can be increased when the client is raising issues that carry a stigma in the prevailing social culture or are strongly associated with social disadvantage in the prevailing social hierarchies. Another pair of challenges may inhibit a client's trust in the counsellor and the counselling processes. They relate to risk and the risk of making changes or the uncertainty of the beneficial outcome of any changes.

It appears to be one of the paradoxes of human experience that the more trapped we are in emotional or mental difficulties, the more frightening it is to imagine the possibility of change.

Trust can be defined as a relationship of sufficient goodwill and resilience to withstand:

- the relational challenges of difference and inequality;
- transitional or existential challenges of risk and uncertainty.

There are many other ways of identifying the key issues involved in trust and mistrust in particular counselling relationships, but probably none are better than discussing them directly with a client when appropriate. Being **trustworthy** as a counsellor requires ethical integrity, **competence**, relational insight supported by good communication skills, and sufficient personal resilience to work with a client's difficulties. This resilience is often enhanced by **supervision** and good relationships with colleagues. Asking ourselves as counsellors what we need to do or be in order to be trustworthy will usually identify significant ethical issues in our work.

Social Justice in Context

Being trustworthy in the face of mistrust requires a strong sense of integrity and resilience. Ed mistrusts his counsellor's wealth and lifestyle that are so different from his own. Imagine yourself in the counsellor's and client's position and consider what are obstacles to trust that will need to be overcome from each person's perspective. What can the counsellor do to increase her trustworthiness? If you are the counsellor, what professional or personal moral qualities/virtues will you draw on?

Challenging unnecessary and counterproductive secrecy between colleagues particularly where that secrecy might conceal unsafe or ineffective practices

Being professionally curious about each other's practice may seem counter-cultural in a profession as concerned about confidentiality and privacy as counselling. However, being professionally curious about each other's practice may be one of the best means of protection that we can offer to our clients against **exploitation** and poor levels of service. Professional curiosity is much more effective than official vetting and barring processes, important as these are. Criminal record checks involved in vetting and barring only identify people who have been detected as criminally exploiting vulnerable people. These are a small minority of cases; in comparison, professional curiosity can be more free-ranging and can identify and deter someone's behaviour before it has reached the level of exploitation (see Chapter 9). Such professional curiosity needs to be respectful of clients and their right to confidentiality whilst taking account of the importance of client safety.

Being constructive and supportive of each other when facing ethical challenges

Finding the courage, resourcefulness and resilience to face ethical challenges is usually much harder when working in isolation. Just as clients are supported by their internalization of a counsellor's goodwill towards them and their opportunities to learn from the counselling process, so can we be supported by the constructive contributions of our peers.

Being willing to challenge each other when we have significant doubts about the safety of someone's practice

A positive professional culture provides both support – as in the previous point – and challenge. Getting the balance right enriches the professional culture and opportunities for learning for everyone. However, there are situations that may arise that will require us to have the courage to raise our concerns about someone's practice with that person. Sometimes this will be sufficient because our concerns will prove ill-founded or adequate countermeasures will have been taken. But where those concerns seem justified and appear to be putting clients at risk of harm, it will be ethically desirable to raise those concerns with an employer or professional body as appropriate. This is much more easily said than done. The history of professions suggests there is a considerable reluctance to challenge each other's practice in this way. It is not unknown for whistleblowers to be treated badly by colleagues even when their concerns have proved more than justified and patients or clients have been protected from significant harm. Although it is reasonable to be cautious about escalating our concerns about the practice of another professional, it is ethically highly desirable that we do so when the need arises.

Ethical Mindfulness

Reason and emotion both have a substantial part to play in being ethical. We need an ability to reason in order to analyse and evaluate our ethical decisions. Emotion helps us to sense what is right or wrong and how it relates to the experience of others. Empathy is the capability to enter imaginatively into the experience of someone and feel how they might feel. It is an essential capability in counselling. But empathy is also the basis of being ethically concerned for others. Feeling and reason combine in ethics in ways that can only be partially or imperfectly captured in words. Each approach to ethics as principles, **values** or virtues, including the relational virtues of care or trust, has strengths and foregrounds some aspect of ethical experience and commitment. But each is also partial and limited. Bond argued that ethical mindfulness transcends these **limitations** in the previous edition of this book. Focusing down on an ethical issue and emptying the mind systematically in order to sense the ethical dynamics at play is a powerful experience. It is a felt sense-making activity – something that blends what is so often separated out. When in touch with a felt sense, our ethical awareness can seem sharper and more grounded. But when that felt sense is elusive, we might feel ethically impoverished, even struggling, detached and purposeless. The first is a state of ethical mindfulness and the second various states of ethical mindlessness. The strength of ethical mindfulness is that sense of being able to dwell on and stay with a challenging ethical issue, feeling its gravity but usually without being overwhelmed. It is possible to move around the issue and experience it from different positions: sometimes the felt sense is verbal but it may not need words. It provides a powerful experience of deepening an appreciation of different aspects of an issue and seeing them afresh in ways that may affirm previous understandings or offer new insights.

Ethical integrity

'Integrity' is a word with many shades of meaning, from being undivided, in a state of completeness, morally upright, sincere or honest. A felt sense is more one of knowing the ground upon which you are standing and a sense of commitment to the wellbeing of another person. Ethical mindfulness does not eliminate the need to use reason and feelings, attempt to communicate in words, or to examine whether good intent produces the desired outcomes: that is one of its limitations. But each of these activities feels as if it represents something of more substance. Something another person can rely on. Ethical mindfulness secures a commitment that is more deeply rooted than reason or feeling alone can achieve. Ethical mindfulness is a state of mind that can be developed and refreshed to help us face the ethical complexity, **diversity** and continually changing nature of contemporary life.

Pause for Reflection

How do you ensure that you are trustworthy to your clients? How trustworthy does your counselling appear to be from a client's perspective? What are the issues that need particular care? Likewise, how do you support other counsellors, particularly colleagues in addressing ethical issues and meeting the challenges of delivering counselling services to an adequate standard?

To access the online resources accompanying this chapter, please visit: https://study.sagepub.com/reevesandbond

Glossary

All terms are defined as currently used in ethics for counselling and the talking therapies.

Acceptance Relating positively to someone's values and identity that may be different from your own.

Accessible Easily entered if a building or space; easy to find and use if an electronic resource.

Accountability Being willing to explain any decisions or actions taken for which you are responsible.

Accredited voluntary register A form of professional regulation in the UK run by the Professional Standards Authority as an alternative to statutory regulation – operates like a kite mark to assure the quality of services offered to the public.

Advice Providing information and an opinion about the best way of acting on that information – the style of advice giving can vary from very directive to facilitative.

Advocacy To give voice in support of another, or of a particular position. Often used in the helping professions to support the cause of someone less able to argue their own case.

Agency policy An agency's preferred course of action that all staff are expected to implement.

Autonomy Ethical principle that protects the right to self-government and to make one's own decisions.

Befriending A way of reaching out to people who are vulnerable or isolated by offering friendship and social support.

Beneficence Ethical principle that prioritizes doing good and benefiting the person affected.

Boundaries The limits between ethically acceptable and unacceptable influence over others or the line between acceptable and unacceptable relationships.

Coaching A type of mentoring that combines modelling and tutoring as ways of improving performance or wellbeing.

Codes Statement of ethical values, principles or rules required to be a member of a particular professional body.

Competence Possessing adequate knowledge and skills in order to perform a task or deliver a service satisfactorily.

Confidentiality Protection of personally sensitive information from unauthorized disclosure. Literally means 'strong trust', i.e. strong enough to be trusted with another person's private information.

Contract An agreement between people about how something will be achieved or delivered – clear contracting strengthens ethical practice.

Counselling 'Counselling' to professional standards means providing knowledgeable, skilled and ethical assistance, typically for emotional, psychological or relational problems. In popular or everyday speech 'counselling' may include giving advice.

Counselling professions A more inclusive of a range of associated activities, such as **counselling**, **psychotherapy**, **counselling skills** and **coaching**, first formally used in BACP's *Ethical Framework for the Counselling Professions*, initially published in 2016.

Counselling skills Skills drawing on the knowledge, skills and ethics of professional counselling to provide informal help to someone in a social context, or used to assist the delivery or as part of a specialized professional role such as nurse, teacher or social worker.

Cultural differences These are differences in values, identity and ways of life between people that need to be taken into account when delivering counselling and deciding what is ethical.

Culture Culture concerns the values, identity and ways of life that influence the ways people interact with each other – an invisible force that can bind people together or seem problematic and puzzling when viewed from another culture.

Digital Involving electronic or computer-generated communications.

Dilemma A difficult choice between two or more options that are similarly good or bad so that there is no obvious preferred choice.

Disability Impaired physical/mental functioning – more positively viewed as 'differently able'. There is an ethical obligation to make reasonable adjustments to empower and enable social inclusion.

Disclosure The communication of personally significant information.

Discrimination Distinguishing between people on the basis of particular characteristics – becomes ethically and legally problematic if it involves treating people in a prejudiced or unfavourable way in comparison to others.

Diversity Being different or varied.

Duty of care A legal term for a personal or social responsibility to someone that forms the basis for liability in negligence when not fulfilled.

Embedded counselling When helpers, including professionals, are willing to listen and respond constructively to the emotional pain and personal stories of people seeking their help.

Equality Where every person has equal rights and a fair chance. It is an approach recognizing that different people have different starting points.

Ethical standards An ethically required level of performance.

Ethics Moral principles or systems of thought to help people distinguish between good and bad.

Euthanasia Enabling a gentle and easy death – a good death.

Evidence-based practice Practice informed by rigorous research into its effectiveness and safety.

Evidence-informed practice Practice informed by a wide range of research approaches beyond randomized controlled trials.

Exploitation Taking unfair advantage of someone.

Guidance Directing someone towards the best possible course of action or decision.

Identity The personal characteristics that enable people to know who they are and what distinguishes them from others.

Illness When good heath is disrupted by infection or other causes.

Impaired functioning Performing at a level below what is usual or desirable for the person affected.

Inclusion Where every person feels respected, valued, and that they have a contribution to make.

Insurance Paying for protection from financial or other types of losses.

Integrity Being honest and actions based on strong moral and ethical principles.

Issues Significant problems or topics that require a decision or action to resolve them.

Justice An ethical and/or legal principle concerning fairness and impartiality.

Law A system of public morals enforced by the courts.

Life-saving treatment Treatments for medical conditions that would otherwise be fatal.

Limitations Restrictions in application or performance.

Mentoring Supportive relationship designed to assist someone with difficult transitions, compensate for disadvantages in their life, or sustain challenging roles.

Mindfulness Consciously brought to the front of your mind and integrated into your sense of self.

Morals Habits of life concerning right and wrong.

Negligence A failure to fulfil a legal duty of care that causes harm.

Non-maleficence Ethical principle that prioritizes 'do no harm' – better to do nothing than to cause harm.

Notes A summary of a counselling session or other professional activities.

Online Communicating with someone by means of the internet, e.g. messaging or video communication.

Practitioner psychologist A legally protected title in the UK that may only be used by someone registered as a specialist psychologist with the Health and Care Professions Council (HCPC).

Prejudice Harm or injury caused by ill-founded judgment of someone.

Privacy Freedom from intrusion or disturbance.

Problems Provokes doubt or causes difficulty.

Process notes Summary of a counsellor's personal feelings and psychological processes in response to a client's communications.

Processing A technical term in data protection for doing just about anything with data.

Psychotherapy *Either* counselling under another name *or* therapy for more severe types of mental illness or personal disturbances.

Public interest For the general good of a community or a nation.

Records Any type of evidence that indicates what happened in counselling.

Regulation Authoritative rule for controlling behaviour or how something ought to be undertaken.

Research A systematic inquiry or experiment to advance knowledge.

Respect Honouring or showing esteem to another person.

Responsibility Commitment to working to an adequate standard for which you are willing to be accountable.

Rights Legally, morally or ethically justified entitlements.

Safety Protected or guarded against harm.

SCoPEd Scope of practice in education and practice in the counselling professions, a project initiated by BACP, UKCP and BPC.

Security Safe from harm or intrusion.

Self-harm Intentionally or recklessly causing injury to self.

Self-respect Treating oneself as worthy of honour and esteem.

Social diversity A description of a social structure that recognizes communities representing difference amongst people, including around age, race, culture, disability, income, gender, sexual identity.

Social media Mass communication using the internet for social purposes.

Standards Recognized level or quality of performance which applies to all services of that type.

Statutory regulation Legal control authorized by government over the entry requirements, standards and discipline for anyone using a specified occupational title.

Suicidal intent A desire to kill oneself.

Suicide The act of killing oneself.

Supervision A type of professional mentoring widely used in the talking therapies to enhance the quality of service provided to clients.

Tolerance Withholding criticism or prejudice but not necessarily offering active support or acceptance.

Trust To have confidence that someone is on your side and doing their best for you.

Trustworthy Behaving in ways in which people, particularly clients, can rely on your goodwill and actions concerning them.

Values What is considered important or good in life.

Voluntary Something undertaken of one's own free will.

References

Adams, M. (2013) *The Myth of the Untroubled Therapist*. Oxford: Routledge.

Aldridge, S. (2014) *A Short Introduction to Counselling*. London: Sage.

Ali, L. and Graham, B. (1996) *The Counselling Approach to Careers Guidance*. London: Taylor & Francis.

American Counseling Association (ACA) (2014) *ACA Code of Ethics*. Alexandria, VA: American Counseling Association.

Amis, K. (2017) *Boundaries, Power and Ethical Responsibility in Counselling and Psychotherapy* (Essential Issues in Counselling and Psychotherapy). London: Sage.

Anthony, K. and Merz Nagel, D. (2015) *Therapy Online [A Practical Guide – Kindle Edition]*. London: Sage.

Argyle, M. (ed.) (1981) *Social Skills and Health*. London: Methuen.

Association for Counselling & Therapy Online (ACTO) (2020) *Professional Conduct and Code of Ethics*. Available at https://acto-org.uk/professional-conduct-code-ethics (accessed July 2020).

Austin, K.M., Moline, M.E. and Williams, G.T. (1990) *Confronting Malpractice: Legal and Ethical Dilemmas in Psychotherapy*. Newbury Park, CA: Sage.

Bacon, F. (2008 [1625]) *The Major Works* (Oxford World Classics), edited by B. Vickers. Oxford: Oxford University Press.

Bancroft, J. (1989) *Human Sexuality and Its Problems*. Edinburgh: Churchill Livingstone.

Banks, S. (2006) *Ethics and Values in Social Work* (3rd edn). Basingstoke: Palgrave Macmillan.

Beauchamp, T.L. and Childress, J.F. (2019) *Principles of Biomedical Ethics* (8th edn). New York: Oxford University Press.

Bond, T. (1989) 'Towards defining the role of counselling skills', *Counselling – Journal of the British Association for Counselling*, 69: 3–9.

Bond, T. (1991) *HIV Counselling – Report on National Survey and Consultation 1990*. Rugby: British Association for Counselling.

Bond, T. (1994) 'Ethical standards and the exploitation of clients', *Counselling – Journal of the British Association for Counselling*, 4 (3), Stop Press: 2–3.

Bond, T. (1997) 'Therapists' dilemmas as stimuli to new understanding and practice', in W. Dryden (ed.), *Therapists' Dilemmas*. London: Sage.

Bond, T. (2006) 'Intimacy, risk, and reciprocity in psychotherapy: intricate ethical challenges', *Transactional Analysis Journal*, 36 (2): 77–89.

Bond, T. (2007) 'Ethics and psychotherapy: an issue of trust', in R.E. Ashcroft, A. Dawson, H. Drapes and J.R. McMillan (eds), *Principles of Health Care Ethics* (2nd edn). Chichester: Wiley.

Bond, T. and Sandhu, A. (2005) *Therapists in Court: Providing Evidence and Supporting Witnesses*. London: Sage.

Brammer, L.M. and Shostrum, E.L. (1982) *Therapeutic Psychology: Fundamentals of Counselling and Psychotherapy*. Englewood Cliffs, NJ: Prentice-Hall.

British Association for Counselling (BAC) (1984) *Code of Ethics and Practice for Counsellors*. Rugby: BAC.

British Association for Counselling (BAC) (1985) *Counselling: Definition of Terms in Use with Expansion and Rationale*. Rugby: BAC.

British Association for Counselling (BAC) (1997) *Code of Ethics and Practice for Counsellors*. Rugby: BAC.

British Association for Counselling and Psychotherapy (BACP) (2008) *What Is Counselling*? Lutterworth: BACP.

British Association for Counselling and Psychotherapy (BACP) (2013) *Ethical Framework for Good Practice in Counselling and Psychotherapy*. Lutterworth: BACP.

British Association for Counselling and Psychotherapy (BACP) (2018a) *Ethical Framework for the Counselling Professions*. Lutterworth: BACP.

British Association for Counselling and Psychotherapy (BACP) (2018b) *Working with Children and Young People within the Counselling Professions: Good Practice in Action 046*. Lutterworth: BACP.

British Association for Counselling and Psychotherapy (BACP) (2019a) *Competencies for Working with Children and Young People (4–18 years)* Lutterworth: BACP.

British Association for Counselling and Psychotherapy (BACP) (2019b) *Working Online in the Counselling Professions: Good Practice in Action 047*. Lutterworth: BACP.

British Association for Counselling and Psychotherapy (BACP) (2020a) *Coaching*. Available at: https://www.bacp.co.uk/bacp-divisions/bacp-coaching

British Association for Counselling and Psychotherapy (BACP) (2020b) *Working with Suicidal Clients in the Counselling Professions: Good Practice in Action 042*. Lutterworth: BACP.

British Psychological Society (BPS) (2017) *Practice Guidelines* (3rd edn). Leicester: BPS.

British Psychological Society (BPS) (2020) *Counselling Psychology*. Available at https://careers.bps.org.uk/area/counselling (accessed October 2020).

Brooke, R. (1972) *Information and Advice Guidance: The Social Administration Research Trust*. London: G. Bell.

Brown, S. (2017) 'Burnout: The high cost of caring?' *Therapy Today*, 28 (9): 3–7.

Caldicott Committee (1997) *Report on the Review of Patient-identifiable Information*. London: Department of Health.

Cameron, R. (2020) *Working with Difference and Diversity in Counselling and Psychotherapy*. London: Sage.

Carroll, M. (1993) 'Ethical issues in organizational counselling'. Unpublished paper, Roehampton Institute, London.

Carroll, M. (2014) *Effective Supervision for the Helping Professions* (2nd edn). London: Sage.

Carroll, M. and Holloway, E. (1999) 'Introduction', in M. Carroll and E. Holloway (eds), *Counselling Supervison in Context*. London: Sage. pp. 1–4.

Carroll, M. and Shaw, E. (2013) *Ethical Maturity in the Helping Professions*. London: Jessica Kingsley.

Central Advisory Council for Education (England) (1963) *Half Our Future*. London: HMSO.

CEOM–ECMO (Conseil européen des Ordres des médecins/European Council of Medical Orders) (2011) http://www.ceom-ecmo.eu/en/view/ethics-charter

Children's Legal Centre (1989) 'A child's right to confidentiality?', *Childright*, 57: 7–10.

Cohen, K. (1992) 'Some legal issues in counselling and psychotherapy', *British Journal of Guidance and Counselling*, 20 (1): 10–26.

College of Sexual and Relationship Therapists (2019) *Good Therapy: CORST Code of Ethics and Practice*. London: CORST.

COSCA (Confederation of Scottish Counselling Agencies) (2014) *Statement of Ethics and Code of Practice*. Stirling: COSCA.

Cooper, M. (2008) *Essential Research Findings in Counselling and Psychotherapy: The Facts Are Friendly*. London: Sage.

Cooper, M. and McLeod, J. (2010) *Pluralistic Counselling and Psychotherapy*. London: Sage.

Cooper, M. and Reeves, A. (2012) 'The role of randomised controlled trials in developing an evidence-base for counselling and psychotherapy', *Counselling and Psychotherapy Research*, 12 (4): 303–7.

Corey, G., Corey, M.S. and Callanan, P. (2003) *Issues and Ethics in the Helping Professions* (6th edn). Pacific Grove, CA: Brooks/Cole.

Council for Healthcare Regulatory Excellence (2008) *Clear Sexual Boundaries between Healthcare Professionals and Patients: Responsibilities of Healthcare Professionals*. London: Council for Healthcare Regulatory Excellence.

Cousins, S. (2019) *Overcoming Everyday Racism: Building Resilience and Wellbeing in the Face of Discrimination and Microaggressions*. London: Jessica Kingsley.

Culley, S. and Bond, T. (2011) *Integrative Counselling skills in Action* (3rd edn). London: Sage.

Dalrymple, J. and Boylan, J. (2013) *Effective Advocacy in Social Work*. London: Sage.

Department of Health (2010) *Confidentiality: NHS Code of Practice*. London: Department of Health.

Dryden, W. (ed.) (1998) *Therapists' Dilemmas* (2nd edn). London: Sage.

Dryden, W. (2020) *The Single-Session Counselling Primer: Principles and Practice*. Monmouth: PCCS Books.

Dryden, W. and Neenan, M. (2004) *Rational Emotive Behavioural Counselling in Action*. London: Sage.

Einzig, H. (1989) *Counselling and Psychotherapy – Is it for Me?* Rugby: British Association for Counselling.

Evans, J. (2009) *Online Counselling and Guidance: A Practical Resource for Trainees and Practitioners*. London: Sage.

Foskett, J. and Lyall, D. (1988) *Helping the Helpers – Supervision and Pastoral Care*. London: SPCK.

Francis, R. (2013) *The Mid-Staffordshire NHS Foundation Trust Public Inquiry*. London: The Stationery Office.

Gabriel, L. (2005) *Speaking the Unspeakable: The Ethics of Dual Relationships in Counselling and Psychotherapy*. London: Routledge.

Gellatly, J., Bower, P., Hennessy, S., Richards, D., Gilbody, S. and Lovell, K. (2007) 'What makes self-help interventions effective in the management of depressive symptoms? Meta-analysis and meta-regression', *Psychological Medicine*, 37: 1217–28.

General Medical Council (2013a) *Doctors' Use of Social Media*. London: GMC.

Giddens, A. (1991) *Modernity and Self Identity: Self and Society in the Late Modern Age*. Cambridge: Polity.

Gillon, R. (1985) 'Autonomy and consent', in M. Lockwood (ed.), *Moral Dilemmas in Modern Medicine*. Oxford: Oxford University Press. pp. 111–25.

Gothard, B., Mignot, P., Offer, M. and Ruff, M. (2001) *Careers Guidance in Context*. London: Sage.

Guardian Law Reports (1992) '*Re J* (a minor) (medical treatment)', *The Guardian*, 22 July.

Gubi, P. (2008) *Prayer in Counselling and Psychotherapy*. London: Jessica Kingsley.

Gubi, P. (2015) *Spiritual Accompaniment and Counselling: Journeying with Psyche and Soul*. London: Jessica Kingsley.

Gubi, P. (2017). *What Counsellors and Spiritual Directors Can Learn from Each Other: Ethical Practice, Training and Supervision*. London: Jessica Kingsley.

Hawkins, P. and Shohet, R. (2012) *Supervison in the Helping Professions* (4th edn). Maidenhead: Open University Press.

Hayman, A. (1965) 'Psychoanalyst subpoenaed', *The Lancet*, 16 October: 785–6.

Health and Care Professions Council (HCPC) (2018) *Standards of Conduct, Performance and Ethics*. London: HCPC.

Herlihy, B. and Corey, G. (1992) *Dual Relationships*. Alexandria, VA: American Association for Counseling and Development.

Heyd, D. and Bloch, S. (1991) 'The ethics of suicide', in S. Bloch and P. Chodoff (eds), *Psychiatric Ethics*. Oxford: Oxford University Press.

Hiltner, S. (1949) *Pastoral Counselling*. Nashville, TN: Abingdon.

HM Government (2018) *Working Together to Safeguard Children*. London: Department for Education.

Holmes, J. and Lindley, R. (1998) *The Values of Psychotherapy*. Oxford: Oxford University Press.

Houston, G. (1995) *Supervision and Counselling* (2nd edn). London: Rochester Foundation.

Human Fertilization & Embryology Authority (HFEA) (2008) *Code of Practice* (8th edn) (Consultation draft). London: HEFA.

Improving Access to Psychological Therapies (IAPT) (2020) *Adult IAPT Programme*. Available at www.england.nhs.uk/mental-health/adults/iapt (accessed August 2020).

Inskipp, F. (1986) *Counselling: The Trainer's Handbook*. Cambridge: National Extension College.

Inskipp, F. and Proctor, B. (1994) *Making the Most of Supervision*. Twickenham: Cascade.

Inskipp, F. and Proctor, B. (1995) *Becoming a Counselling Supervisor*. Twickenham: Cascade.

International Association for Counselling (IAC) (2003) *Who We Are*. London: IAC, and Paris: UNESCO.

Irish Association for Counselling and Psychotherapy (IACP) (2018) *Code of Ethics and Practice*. Bray: IACP.

Jacobs, M. (2010) *Psychodynamic Counselling in Action* (4th edn). London: Sage.

Jakobi, S. and Pratt, D. (1992) 'Therapy note and the law', *The Psychologist*, May: 219–21.

Jehu, D. (1994) *Patients as Victims: Sexual Abuse in Psychotherapy and Counselling*. Chichester: Wiley.

Jenkins, P. (1996) *False or Recovered Memories? Legal and Ethical Implications for Therapists*. London: Sage.

Jenkins, P. (2007) *Counselling, Psychotherapy and the Law* (2nd edn). London: Sage.

Jenkins, P. (2012) *Legal Issues in Counselling and Psychotherapy* (online version). London: Sage.

Jones, G. and Stokes, A. (2009) *Online Counselling*. Houndsmill: Palgrave Macmillan.

Kaplan, D.M. (2014) 'Ethical implications of a critical legal case for the counseling profession: Ward v Wilbanks', *Journal of Counseling and Development*, 92: 142–6.

Khele, S., Symons, C. and Wheeler, S. (2008) 'An analysis of complaints to the British Association for Counselling and Psychotherapy 1996–2006', *Counselling and Psychotherapy Research*, 8 (2): 124–32.

Lago, C. (2008) *Race, Culture and Counselling: The Ongoing Challenge* (2nd edn). Milton Keynes: Open University Press.

Lago, C. and Smith, B. (2010) *Anti-Discriminatory Practice in Counselling and Psychotherapy* (2nd edn). London: Sage.

Laing, R.D. (1967) *The Politics of Experience and the Bird of Paradise*. Harmondsworth: Penguin.

Laungani, P. (2004) *Asian Perspectives in Counselling and Psychotherapy*. Hove: Brunner-Routledge.

Law Commission (1981) *Breach of Confidence*. Cmnd 8388. London: HMSO.

Layard, R., Clark, D., Knapp, M. and Mayraz, G. (2007) 'Cost–benefit analysis of psychological therapy', *National Institute Economic Review*, 202: 90–98.

Lynch, G. (2002) *Pastoral Care and Counselling*. London: Sage.

Mackenzie, C. and Stoljar, N. (2000) *Relational Autonomy: Feminist Perspectives on Autonomy, Agency and the Social Self*. Oxford: Oxford University Press.

Mason, R. and Reeves, A. (2018) 'An exploration of how working in the Improving Access to Psychological Therapies (IAPT) programme might affect the personal and professional development of counsellors: an analytical autoethnographic study', *British Journal of Guidance and Counselling*, 46 (6): 669–78.

Masson, J. (1985) *The Assault on Truth*. Harmondsworth: Penguin.

McKenzie-Mavinga, I. (2009) *Black Issues in the Therapeutic Process*. Basingstoke: Palgrave Macmillan.

McLeod, J. (1997) *Narrative and Psychotherapy*. London: Sage.

McLeod, J. (1998) *An Introduction to Counselling* (2nd edn). Buckingham: Open University Press.

McLeod, J. and McLeod, J. (2011) *Counselling Skill* (2nd edn). Maidenhead: Open University Press.

Mearns, D., Thorne, B. and McLeod, J. (2013) *Person-Centred Counselling in Action* (4th edn). London: Sage.

Mental Health Apps NHS (2020) *Mental Health Apps*. Available at www.nhs.uk/apps-library/category/mental-health (accessed August 2020).

Mill, J. (1859) *On Liberty*. Ontario: Batoche Books Limited. Available at https://socialsciences.mcmaster.ca/econ/ugcm/3ll3/mill/liberty.pdf (accessed November 2020).

Miller, A. (1998) *Thou Shalt Not Be Aware*. London: Pluto.

Mitchels, B. (2006) *Love in Danger: Trauma, Therapy and Conflict Explored through the Life and Work of Adam Curle*. Charlbury: John Carpenter.

Mitchels, B. and Bond, T. (2010) *Essential Law for Counsellors and Psychotherapists*. London: Sage.

Mitchels, B. and Bond, T. (2011) *Legal Issues across Counselling and Psychotherapy Settings*. London: Sage.

Mitchels, B. and Bond, T. (2021) *Confidentiality & Record Keeping in Counselling & Psychotherapy* (3rd edn). London: Sage.

Moodley, R. and West, W. (eds) (2005) *Integrating Traditional Healing into Counseling and Psychotherapy*. Thousand Oaks, CA: Sage.

National Institute for Health and Care Excellence (NICE) (2009) *Depression: The Treatment and Management of Depression in Adults*. NICE guideline 90. London: NICE.

National Institute for Health and Care Excellence (NICE) (2011) *Self-harm: Longer-term Management*. NICE guidelines (CG133). London: NICE.

New Zealand Association of Counsellors (NZAC) (1998) 'Code of ethics', in *New Zealand Association of Counsellors Handbook 1998*. Auckland: NZAC.

New Zealand Association of Counsellors (NZAC) (2020) *Code of Ethics: A Framework for Ethical Practice 2002* (revised 2020). Wellington: NZAC.

O'Connor, R.C. (2010) 'Psychological perspectives on suicidal behaviour', in U. Kumar and M.K. Mandal (eds), *Suicidal Behaviour: Assessment of People at Risk*. New Delhi: Sage.

Page, S. and Wosket, V. (2014) *Supervising the Counsellor: A Cyclical Model* (3rd edn). London: Routledge.

Paradise, L.V. and Siegelwaks, B. (1982) 'Ethical training for group leaders', *Journal for Specialists in Groupwork*, 7 (3): 162–6.

Pedersen, P., Draguns, J.G., Lonner, W.J. and Trimble, J.E. (2008) *Counselling across Cultures* (6th edn). Thousand Oaks, CA: Sage.

Ponterotto, J.G., Casas, J.M., Suzuki, L.A. and Alexander, C.M. (eds) (2009) *Handbook of Multicultural Counseling* (3rd edn). Thousand Oaks, CA: Sage.

Pope, K.S. (1988) 'How clients are harmed by sexual contact with mental health professionals: the syndrome and its prevalence', *Journal of Counseling and Development*, 67: 222–6.

Pope, K.S. and Bouhoutsos, J.C. (1986) *Sexual Intimacy between Therapists and Patients*. New York: Praeger.

Pope, K.S. and Vasquez, M.J.T. (1991) *Ethics in Psychotherapy and Counseling: A Practical Guide for Psychologists*. San Francisco, CA: Jossey-Bass.

Pope, K.S., Sonne, J.L. and Greene, B. (2006) *What Therapists Don't Talk about and Why: Understanding Taboos That Hurt Us and Our Clients*. Washington, DC: American Psychological Association.

Proctor, B. (1988) 'Supervision: a co-operative exercise in accountability', in M. Marken and M. Payne (eds), *Enabling and Ensuring Supervision in Practice*. Leicester: National Youth Bureau.

Psychotherapy and Counselling Federation of Australia (PACFA) (2011) *Code of Ethics: The Ethical Framework for Best Practice in Counselling and Psychotherapy*. North Fitzroy: PACFA.

Psychotherapy and Counselling Federation of Australia (PACFA) (2020) https://www.pacfa.org.au/about/mission-values

Pybis, J., Saxon, D., Hill, A. and Barkham, M. (2017) 'The comparative effectiveness and efficiency of cognitive behaviour therapy and generic counselling in the treatment of depression: evidence from the 2nd UK National Audit of psychological therapies', *BMC Psychiatry*, 17 (215).

Reeves, A. (2010) *Counselling Suicidal Clients*. London: Sage.

Reeves, A. (2015) *Working with Risk in Counselling and Psychotherapy*. London: Sage.

Reeves, A. (2018) *An Introduction to Counselling and Psychotherapy: From Theory to Practice* (2nd edn). London: Sage.

Reiter-Theil, S., Eich, H. and Reiter, L. (1991) 'Informed consent in family therapy – necessary discourse and practice', *Changes: an International Journal of Psychology and Psychotherapy*, 9 (2): 91–100.

Rogers, J. (2012) *Coaching Skills: A Handbook*. New York: McGraw Hill, Open University Press .

Rogers, W.V.H. (2010) *Winfield and Jolowicz on Tort* (18th edn). London: Sweet & Maxwell.

Rowan, J. (1988) 'Counselling and the psychology of furniture', *Counselling – Journal of the British Association for Counselling*, 64: 21–45.

Russell, J. (1993) *Out of Bounds: Sexual Exploitation in Counselling and Therapy*. London: Sage.

Russell, J. (1996) 'Sexual exploitation in counselling in future developments in counselling', in R. Bayne, I. Horton and J. Bimrose (eds), *New Directions in Counselling*. London: Routledge. pp. 65–78.

Rutter, P. (1989) *Sex in the Forbidden Zone*. London: Mandala.

Sackett, D. (1996) 'Evidence-based medicine – what it is and what it isn't', *British Medical Journal*, 312: 71–2.

Sanders, P. and Hill, A. (2014) *Counselling for Depression: A Person-centred and Experiential Approach to Practice*. London: Sage.

SCoPEd (2020a) SCoPEd *Framework: A Draft Framework for the Practice and Education of Counselling and Psychotherapy*. London: BACP, UKCP and BPC.

SCoPEd (2020b) *A Framework for Counselling and Psychotherapy*. Available at www.bacp.co.uk/about-us/advancing-the-profession/scoped (accessed September 2020).

Scottish Intercollegiate Guidelines Network (SIGN) (2010) *Non-pharmaceutical Management of Depression in Adults: National Clinical Guidelines*. Edinburgh: SIGN.

Silverman, D. (1996) *Discourses of Counselling: HIV Counselling as Social Interaction*. London: Sage.

Sommers-Flanagan, R. and Sommers-Flanagan, J. (2007) *Becoming an Ethical Helping Professional: Cultural and Philosophical Foundations*. Hoboken, NJ: Wiley.

Southern Derbyshire Health Authority (SDHA) (1996) *Report of the Inquiry into the Care of Anthony Smith*. Derby: Southern Derbyshire Health Authority and Derbyshire County Council.

Stadler, H.A. (1986a) *Confidentiality: The Professional's Dilemma – Participant Manual*. Alexandria, VA: American Association for Counseling and Development.

Stadler, H.A. (1986b) 'Making hard choices: clarifying controversial ethical issues', *Counseling and Human Development*, 19 (1): 1–10.

Stewart, D. (2014) 'Appraising internet self help', *Healthcare Counselling and Psychotherapy Journal*, April: 24–6.

Stokes, A. (2018) *Online Supervision: A Handbook for Practitioners*. London: Routledge.

Stoltenberg, C.D. and Delworth, U. (1987) *Supervising Counselors and Therapists: A Developmental Approach*. San Francisco, CA: Jossey-Bass.

Syme, G. (2003) *Dual Relationships in Counselling and Psychotherapy: Exploring the Limits*. London: Sage.

Szasz, T. (1986) 'The case against suicide prevention', *American Psychologist*, 41: 806–12.

Thompson, A. (1990) *A Guide to Ethical Practice in Psychotherapy*. New York: Wiley.

Thorne, B. (1992) 'Psychotherapy and counselling: the quest for differences', *Counselling – Journal of the British Association for Counselling*, 3 (4): 244–8.

Trower, P., Casey, A. and Dryden, W. (2011) *Cognitive-Behavioural Counselling in Action* (2nd edn). London: Sage.

United Kingdom Council for Psychotherapy (UKCP) (2019) *UKCP Ethical Principles and Code of Professional Conduct*. London: UKCP.

Weinberg, H. and Rolnick, A. (2019) *Theory and Practice of Online Therapy*. Oxford: Routledge.

Weitz, P. (ed.) (2014) *Psychotherapy 2.0*. London: Karnac.

Wheeler, S. and Richards, K. (2007) *The Impact of Clinical Supervision on Counsellors and Therapists, Their Practice and Their Clients: A Systematic Review of the Literature*. Lutterworth: BACP.

Wise, C. (1951) *Pastoral Counseling: Its Theory and Practice*. New York: Harper.

Index

CPSIA information can be obtained
at www.ICGtesting.com
Printed in the USA
JSHW050453100722
27894JS00003B/248

9 781526 458865